Dementia in Clinical Practice

Frontiers of Neurology and Neuroscience

Vol. 24

Series Editor

J. Bogousslavsky Montreux

Dementia in Clinical Practice

Volume Editors

P. Giannakopoulos Geneva

P.R. Hof New York, N.Y.

15 figures, 2 in color, and 17 tables, 2009

KARGER

Basel · Freiburg · Paris · London · New York · Bangalore · Bangkok · Shanghai · Singapore · Tokyo · Sydney

Prof. Panteleimon Giannakopoulos
Division of Geriatric Psychiatry
Department of Psychiatry
University of Geneva School of Medicine
2, chemin du Petit-Bel-Air
CH–1225 Chêne-Bourg, Geneva (Switzerland)

Prof. Patrick R. Hof
Regenstreif Professor of Neuroscience
Vice-Chair, Department of Neuroscience
Kastor Neurobiology of Aging Laboratories
Mount Sinai School of Medicine
New York, NY 10029 (USA)

Library of Congress Cataloging-in-Publication Data
Dementia in clinical practice / volume editors, P. Giannakopoulos, P.R . Hof.
p. ; cm. -- (Frontiers of neurology and neuroscience, ISSN 1660-4431
; v. 24)
Includes bibliographical references and indexes.
ISBN 978-3-8055-9015-0 (hard cover : alk. paper)
1. Dementia. I. Giannakopoulos, P. (Panteleimon) II. Hof, Patrick R. III.
Series: Frontiers of neurology and neuroscience ; v. 24.
[DNLM: 1. Dementia--diagnosis. 2. Dementia--therapy. 3. Diagnostic
Imaging--methods. WM 220 D376374 2009]
RC521.D4555 2009
616. 8'3--dc22

2008052906

Bibliographic Indices. This publication is listed in bibliographic services, including Current Contents® and Index Medicus.

www.karger.com
Printed in Switzerland on acid-free and non-aging paper (ISO 9706) by Reinhardt Druck, Basel
ISSN 1660–4431
ISBN 978–3–8055–9015–0
e-ISBN 978–3–8055–9016–7

Contents

List of Contributors

Frédéric Assal
Faculty of Medicine and Neurology
Department of Clinical Neurosciences
University Hospitals of Geneva
rue du Micheli-du-Crest 24
CH–1211 Geneva (Switzerland)

Constantin Bouras
Division of Neuropsychiatry
Department of Psychiatry
University of Geneva Hospitals
2, chemin du Petit-Bel-Air
CH–1225 Chêne-Bourg, Geneva (Switzerland)

Marie-Pierre Deiber
INSERM U877, Faculty of Medicine
FR–38706 La Tronche Cedex (France)

Leonardo C. de Souza
INSERM 610, Pavillion Claude Bernard
Hôpital de la Pitié-Salpêtrière
47, Boulevard de l'Hôpital
FR–75651 Paris Cedex 13 (France)

Bruno Dubois
INSERM-UPMC UMRS 610
Federation of Neurology AP-HP
Hôpital de la Salpêtrière
47-83, Boulevard de l'Hôpital
FR–75013 Paris (France)

Timo Erkinjuntti
Memory Research Unit, Department of Neurology
Helsinki University Central Hospital
PO Box 300
FI–00029 Helsinki (Finland)

Serge Gauthier
McGill Center for Studies in Aging
6825 LaSalle Blvd.
Montréal, QC, H4H 1R3 (Canada)

Panteleimon Giannakopoulos
Division of Geriatric Psychiatry
Department of Psychiatry
University of Geneva School of Medicine
2, chemin du Petit-Bel-Air
CH–1225 Chêne-Bourg, Geneva (Switzerland)

Celine Goetz
Pritzker School of Medicine
University of Chicago
5458 S. Cornell Ave.
Chicago, IL 60615 (USA)

Gabriel Gold
Department of Geriatrics and Rehabilitation
Hôpital des Trois-Chênes
3, chemin du Pont-Bochet,
CH–1226 Thônex, Geneva (Switzerland)

Patrick R. Hof
Regenstreif Professor of Neuroscience
Department of Neuroscience
Kastor Neurobiology of Aging Laboratories
Mount Sinai School of Medicine
New York, NY 10029 (USA)

Vicente Ibáñez
Neuroimaging Unit
Department of Psychiatry
2, chemin du Petit-Bel-Air
CH–1225 Chêne-Bourg, Geneva (Switzerland)

Kurt A. Jellinger
Institute of Clinical Neurobiology
Kenyongasse 18
AT–1070 Vienna (Austria)

Andrew Kertesz
University of Western Ontario
St. Joseph's Hospital
268 Grosvenor St.
London, ON, N6A 4V2 (Canada)

Enikö Kövari
Division of Neuropsychiatry
Department of Psychiatry
Geneva School of Medicine
2, chemin du Petit-Bel-Air
CH–1225 Chêne-Bourg, Geneva (Switzerland)

Mario F. Mendez
Neurobehavior Unit (116AF)
V.A. Greater Los Angeles Healthcare System
11301 Wilshire Blvd.
Los Angeles, CA 90073 (USA)

Reto Meuli
Department of Radiology and
Interventional Radiology
Centre Hospitalier Universitaire
Vaudois and University of Lausanne
CH–1011 Lausanne (Switzerland)

Agnès Michon
Psychiatry Department, Division of
Geriatric Psychiatry
University Hospitals of Geneva (HUG)
2, chemin du Petit-Bel-Air
CH–1225 Chêne-Bourg, Geneva (Switzerland)

Pascal Missonnier
Neuroimaging Unit, Department of
Psychiatry
University of Geneva Hospitals
2, chemin du Petit-Bel-Air
CH–1225 Chêne-Bourg, Geneva (Switzerland)

Agneta Nordberg
Karolinska Institutet, Department of
Neurobiology
Care Sciences and Society, Division of
Alzheimer Neurobiology
Karolinska University Hospital
Huddinge, Novum 5th floor
SE–141 86 Stockholm (Sweden)

Leonardo Pantoni
Department of Neurological and
Psychiatric Sciences
University of Florence
Viale Morgagni 85
IT–50134 Florence (Italy)

Anna Poggesi
Deparment of Neurological and
Psychiatric Sciences
University of Florence
Viale Morgagni 85
IT–50134 Florence (Italy)

Marie Sarazin
Fédération des Maladies du Système
Nerveux
Research and Resource Memory Centre,
Pavillon Paul Castaigne
Hôpital de la Salpêtrière
47, Boulevard de l'Hôpital
FR–75013 Paris (France)

William W. Seeley
University of California, San Francisco
UCSF Memory and Aging Center, Box 1207
San Francisco, CA 94143-1207 (USA)

Marian van der Meulen
Faculty of Medicine and Neurology
Department of Clinical Neurosciences
University Hospitals of Geneva
rue du Micheli-du-Crest 24
CH–1211 Geneva (Switzerland)

Armin von Gunten
Service de Psychiatrie de l'Age Avancé
(SUPAA)
Département de Psychiatrie
Centre Hospitalier Universitaire Vaudois
and University of Lausanne
Route du Mont
CH–1008 Prilly (Switzerland)

Dina Zekry
Hôpital des Trois-Chênes
3, chemin du Pont-Bochet
CH–1226 Thônex, Geneva (Switzerland)

Preface

Research on dementing illnesses is in the midst of an agitated period. During the past 50 years, it has progressively matured from a primarily social service problem to the clinicopathological definition of a wide spectrum of diseases, evaluation of measures of cognition, analysis of brain microstructure, and, more recently, visualization of the pathological substrates such as b-amyloid and tau protein in vivo. Despite these impressive developments in diagnostic tools, biomarkers, and imaging modalities, we still ignore the etiology of the more frequent clinical syndromes leading to the irreversible loss of cognitive functions, namely Alzheimer's disease, Lewy body disease, vascular and frontotemporal dementia. Recent epidemiological work highlights the complex relationships among these entities by demonstrating the high frequency of mixed conditions in very old people and indicating that they may share common risk factors. Moreover, the old and still unresolved question of the limits between normal and pathological aging is to date complicated not only by the description of several transitional forms of mild cognitive impairment characterized by the predominance of brain compensation phenomena that allow for preserving cognitive performances and social adaptation despite an often substantial biological compromise but also by poor response to currently available substitution treatments. Paralleling the difficulty to formulate clear pathogenetic hypotheses, an accelerated pace of compounds entering clinical trials are now available mainly for Alzheimer's disease. Most agents still target clinical end points associated with mild to moderate forms of the disease rather than focus on modulation of the underlying pathologies. Although there are obvious practical but also ethical reasons for this, meaningful progress in other areas of medicine such as cardiology and oncology has targeted and monitored improvement or abatement of pathology as the primary end point as a successful disease-modifying strategy.

In this rather uncertain context, new evidences from basic and clinical sciences should be available in a simple and comprehensive form for general practitioners and mental health professionals. In fact, the pivotal role of clinicians assuming the day-to-day hard work with demented patients and their families may be reinforced by a better integration of current knowledge in the field of dementia pathogenesis, diagnostic procedures and therapeutic possibilities. Avoiding an overspecialized approach, this book aims to provide such an updated view of the disorders likely to be encountered in a daily practice and reviews the major issues presented by each clinical entity in terms of disease pathophysiology, overlap of conditions, diagnosis, therapeutic possibilities and recommendations about patient management issues. To facilitate reading for a nonspecialist, each section is focused on a major form of dementia and is organized following the same scheme reviewing the pathophysiology of the disease, its diagnostic challenges, its characteristic neuroimaging features, and therapeutic interventions. We also hope that this book will reach an additional goal, that of bridging the gap between clinical practice, advanced imaging, recent therapeutics, and basic sciences in order to be an excellent guide for mental health professionals working in the field of dementia.

Panteleimon Giannakopoulos
Patrick R. Hof

Giannakopoulos P, Hof PR (eds): Dementia in Clinical Practice.
Front Neurol Neurosci. Basel, Karger, 2009, vol 24, pp 1–11

Clinical Investigations in Primary Care

Leonardo Cruz de Souza · Marie Sarazin · Celine Goetz · Bruno Dubois

Research and Resource Memory Centre, INSERM UMR S-610, Université Pierre et Marie Curie – Paris 06, Pitié-Salpêtrière Hospital, Paris, France

Abstract

Alzheimer's disease (AD) is a progressive neurodegenerative disorder that represents the most common form of dementia. The most prominent feature of AD is the decline in cognitive function, with an early impairment of episodic memory. The memory deficit of an AD patient is characterized by the amnestic syndrome of the medial temporal type. As the disease progresses, the condition often manifests in language disorders, visuospatial deficits and executive dysfunctions. Patients often have neuropsychiatric disturbances, as apathy and psychotic symptoms. Loss of autonomy follows cognitive impairment. The clinical diagnosis of AD is based on a complete medical examination with a neuropsychological evaluation. The FCSRT (free and cued selective reminding test) is recommended for the identification of the amnestic syndrome of the medial temporal type, which is defined by: (1) a very poor free recall and (2) a decreased total recall due to an insufficient effect of cueing. The neuropsychological tests should also assess other cognitive functions that may be perturbed in AD, such as executive functions, praxis, visuospatial capacities and language. Neuroimaging and biological exams (genetics, biomarkers) are of great utility in the evaluation. Other medical, neurological, or psychiatric disorders which could account for the impairment in memory and related symptoms must be always investigated.

As life expectancy increases, so does the prevalence of dementia: more than one third of individuals over the age of 80 are likely to develop dementia [1]. Alzheimer's disease (AD) is a progressive neurodegenerative disorder that remains the most common cause of dementia [1] and accounts for 50–60% of all cases [2]. Although AD mainly affects aged populations, it should be noted that it also affects an important group of young patients [3].

The stage at which diagnosis is made impacts the therapy advised, the counseling given to patients and family, and the approach to long-term care.

Clinical Features

Progression of Cognitive Deficits Follows the Progression of the Underlying Cerebral Lesions

The most prominent feature of AD is the decline in cognitive function [4]. Memory impairment of recent events, unusual repeated omissions, and difficulty learning new information characterize the first clinical signs. At early stages, when signs are primarily limited to memory impairment, the diagnosis can be difficult and expert advice is often necessary. As the disease progresses, the condition often manifests in language disorders, visuospatial deficits and difficulties executing more complex tasks of daily living.

With regards to anosognosia (loss of insight into cognitive difficulties), some studies suggest that insight is preserved in the early stages of the disease but then diminishes as the condition progresses [4]. However, it is often the family who initiates consultation rather than the patient.

Loss of autonomy follows cognitive impairment. Patients progress from loss of higher-level activities of daily living, such as financial transactions and the use of public transportation, to abnormalities in the more basic activities of daily living.

This progression of cognitive deficits is related to the progression of the underlying cerebral lesions [1], as established by Braak and Braak [5]. In the early stages of AD (Braak I–III), critical areas for episodic memory are already effected by neuropathological changes (neurofibrillary degeneration) in medial temporal regions (hippocampal formations, parahippocampal gyrus, and entorhinal cortex) and, consequently, episodic memory deficit is the initial and reliable neuropsychological marker of AD. As the condition progresses, deficits occur in instrumental functions (language, praxis, visuospatial capacities), which are consistent with the extension of lesions into the neocortical association areas (Braak V).

Amnesic Syndrome Is the Main Symptom

Not all aspects of memory are equally affected in early AD; impairment of anterograde episodic memory tends to be the initial and most prominent indicator [4, 6].

A specific pattern of low performance during memory testing is required for AD diagnosis. The FCSRT (free and cued selective reminding test) [7] is recommended for evaluation of an undiagnosed patient [8], because poor information storage as evident with a low total recall performance after facilitation of retrieval by semantic cues [9] characterizes the typical profile of AD memory deficit (so-called amnestic syndrome of the medial temporal type).

Poor memory performances can be observed in other medical disorders such as Parkinson disease with dementia, vascular dementia, depression, and iatrogenic mechanism. Moreover, subjective memory complaints are common in the aging population. The perceptions of patients' symptoms from a proxy are perhaps more reliable as they often reflect an objective perspective on memory performance.

Temporal-Spatial Disorientation

Temporal-spatial disorientation (disorientation in nonfamiliar places and difficulty recalling recent events) characterizes the earliest stages of the disease [6]. Patients often report difficulty orienting themselves in familiar places (neighborhood) during intermediate stages and progress to severe disorientation in their personal residence in later stages.

Instrumental Cognitive Functions Deficit

In early stages, patients may have normal language abilities. Aphasia (language disorders) may appear as the condition progresses, marked by decreased verbal comprehension and naming difficulty [6]. Some patients may present with aphasia at the onset. During picture-naming tasks, the patient will use nonspecific words (e.g. 'trick', 'thing') periphrases, or words belonging to a superordered category ('fruit' for 'banana') or the same category ('apple' for 'pear'). As AD advances, language disorders can severely impair comprehension, reading and writing, resulting in mutism or incomprehensible language [6]. Clinicians should evaluate whether the patient's discourse is fluent and meaningful, whether simple or complex commands are easily understood, and whether words are lacking during a picture naming task.

Gestural apraxia refers to an inability to perform learned skilled movements, which can not be explained by sensitive motor deficits or by judgment alteration. It is usually measured by asking the patient to perform pantomimes of tool uses (e.g. asking the patient to imitate how to cut with scissors), symbolic gestures (asking the patient to perform a military salute) or to imitate meaningless gestures. At early stages of the disease, gestural apraxia may have little clinical impact on everyday life and accordingly, it must be specifically investigated during the clinical examination. Difficulty using objects, as well as dressing apraxia, is observed during moderate to severe AD.

Visuospatial dysfunction tends to be common in the moderate stage of AD [4]. Deficits arise first during complex tasks, which require perceptual analysis and spatial planning. Impairment in constructional ability can be easily tested by drawing and copying tasks. Occasionally, visuospatial dysfunction dominates early in the so-called visual variant of AD [4].

Visual agnosia and complex visual processing dysfunction are observed in advanced stages of the disease. Patients are impaired in their recognition of objects or faces.

Working Memory and Executive Function

Executive function refers to high-order cognitive abilities that are required for selecting and monitoring appropriate sequence of actions for elaborating goal-directed behaviors [10].

The executive function of working memory (WM) is involved in consecutive processing and information maintenance, and requires attentional resources. Deficits in WM and in attention are not specific, but by the time most patients are diagnosed with established AD, these deficits are usually apparent [4]. Clinicians may observe a decrease in forward and backward digit span or mental ordering. Mental calculation, as tested in the Mini-Mental Test Examination (MMSE), can be disturbed by WM deficits. There is evidence that the attentional and WM deficits are explained not only by an alteration to the dorsolateral prefrontal cortex, but also by a loss of functional integrity of the hippocampal-based memory system which is directly related to alterations of neural activity in parietal regions seen over the course of mild cognitive impairment (MCI) and AD [11].

Executive functions also involve conceptualization and abstract thinking. These abilities can be clinically explored with tests of similarities ('consider a banana and an orange: in what way are they alike?'), tests of differences ('consider a river and a canal: in what way are they not alike?'), or by explanations of proverbs and definitions of symbolic concepts.

The Frontal Assessment Battery [10] is a rapid and efficient tool for assessing frontal (executive) functions in clinical practice.

Severity of the Disease

Different stages of severity are described in AD, from mild to moderate and severe. The Clinical Dementia Rating Score [12] is based on an overall evaluation of the patient's condition and offers incremental stages of severity.

The MMSE [13] assesses the global cognitive efficiency and can discern the level of dementia severity. While the MMSE is not a good test for definitive AD diagnosis, it is easy and quick to administer and can track the overall progression of cognitive decline. Longitudinal studies have shown that the mean annual rate of progression of cognitive impairment using MMSE is approximately 2–6 points [14].

Functional decline increases with disease progression. In mild stages of AD, patients require limited home care. In moderate stages, patients need supervision and regular assistance in most activities. In severe stages, residential health care is necessary.

Neuropsychiatric Symptoms and Behavioral Disturbances

Behavioral and psychological symptoms of dementia include depression, apathy, agitation, aggressivity, and sleep disruption, as well as psychotic symptoms, such as delusions and hallucinations.

The levels of behavioral and psychological symptoms of dementia, especially those of psychosis, depression, and agitation, tend to fluctuate over time, resulting in distinct individual differences. In spite of this variation, it should be noted that the prevalence of psychosis and behavioral disturbance increases as the disease progresses and may indicate a poor prognosis [15].

The most prominent behavioral symptom is apathy, which has been found in 25–50% of cases [4]. It is of note that apathy should not be confounded with depression, as half of AD patients with apathy have no concomitant depression [4]. The prevalence of apathy increases with the severity of dementia. Starkstein et al. [16]

showed that apathy is a behavioral feature of a more aggressive dementia with faster progression of cognitive, functional and emotional impairment.

Delusions are observed more often than hallucinations – their frequency is estimated at 20–70% [4]. Paranoid delusions are probably the most common type, but misidentification phenomena and Capgras delusions may also be observed. Hallucinations, usually visual, are rare in the early stages, but become more prevalent as the disease progresses [4].

Physical Examination

Motor signs on clinical examination are relatively uncommon at the initial stages of AD. Any neurological sign, such as an extrapyramidal syndrome, gait disorders, movement disorders, myoclonus, seizures, lead to discussion of other diagnoses. These features are uncommon until the late phases of the disease.

Some mild motor symptoms can be observed in the latter course of AD. These symptoms consist of changes in muscular tonus (hypertonia, paratonia), cogwheel phenomenon, postural instability and gait disorders, myoclonus, etc. Although characterized under the general term of 'extrapyramidal signs,' these motor symptoms never comprise a true parkinsonian syndrome, which typically consists of unilateral onset, akineto-rigid syndrome, and resting tremor with a good response to levodopa. Scarmeas et al. [17] showed that tremor and bradykinesia motor signs predict cognitive and functional decline, institutionalization, and mortality in AD patients.

Myoclonus may appear later in the course of the disease [6]. Myoclonus is also a significant predictor of functional impairment and it is ultimately a predictor of disease course and death.

Physical examination should always include assessment of vascular risk factors and nutrition.

Diagnosis Criteria

For more than 20 years, the diagnosis of AD has been based on the NINCDS-ADRDA criteria [18], according to which the diagnosis is classified as definite (clinical diagnosis with histological confirmation), probable (typical clinical syndrome without histological confirmation), or possible (atypical clinical features but no alternative diagnosis apparent; no histological confirmation). Typical sensitivity and specificity values for the diagnosis of probable AD with the use of these criteria are 0.81 and 0.73, respectively [19]. In 2007, new diagnostic criteria [8] proposed no more reference to dementia threshold.

To meet the criteria for probable AD, an affected individual must fulfill the core clinical criterion: objective evidence of significantly impaired memory upon testing, and at least one or more of the supportive biological features, including presence of medial temporal lobe atrophy, abnormal cerebrospinal biomarkers, and specific functional neuroimaging patterns with PET. A definite diagnosis of AD can only be made by neuropathology analysis or by both clinical and genetic evidence of AD.

Investigations for Diagnosis

Neuropsychological Assessment

A medical history accompanied by clinical, neurological, and psychiatric examination serves as the foundation for the diagnostic workup. The neuropsychological evaluation is crucial to establishing the nature of memory impairment and remains the cornerstone for diagnosis [8].

Neuropsychological testing can provide objective evidence of and help quantify the precise nature of the memory deficit, especially in the early stages of the disease when other diagnoses may be considered, such as depression. One of the dilemmas in early AD diagnosis is how to distinguish real memory impairment (e.g. failure of information storage and new memory creation) from attentional disorders or strategic impairment (such as normal aging or frontal disorders; fig. 1). In order to characterize the amnestic disorders of an individual suspected of AD, the FCSRT is recommended [8], because it can identify the amnesic syndrome of the medial temporal type, defined by: (1) a very poor free recall and (2) a decreased total recall due to an insufficient effect of cueing. The low performance of total recall in spite of retrieval facilitation indicates a poor storage of information. This amnestic syndrome of the medial temporal type differs from functional and subcortico-frontal memory disorders, which are characterized by a low free recall performance with normal total recall because of good cueing efficacy [20].

The amnestic syndrome of the medial temporal type is able to distinguish patients at an early stage of AD from MCI nonconverters [21].

The neuropsychological test should also assess other cognitive functions that may be perturbed in AD, such as executive functions, praxis, visuospatial capacities and language.

Laboratory Studies

Laboratory studies are necessary to identify or rule out secondary causes of dementia and coexisting disorders that are common in elderly people. The following tests are recommended for evaluation: complete blood cell count, glucose, thyroid function tests, serum electrolytes, BUN/creatine, serum B_{12} levels, liver function tests [22]. Screening for syphilis and serology for HIV should be considered in selected patients.

Lumbar puncture should be acquired for patients younger than 55 years old, in cases of rapidly progressing or unusual dementia, hydrocephalus, immunosuppression,

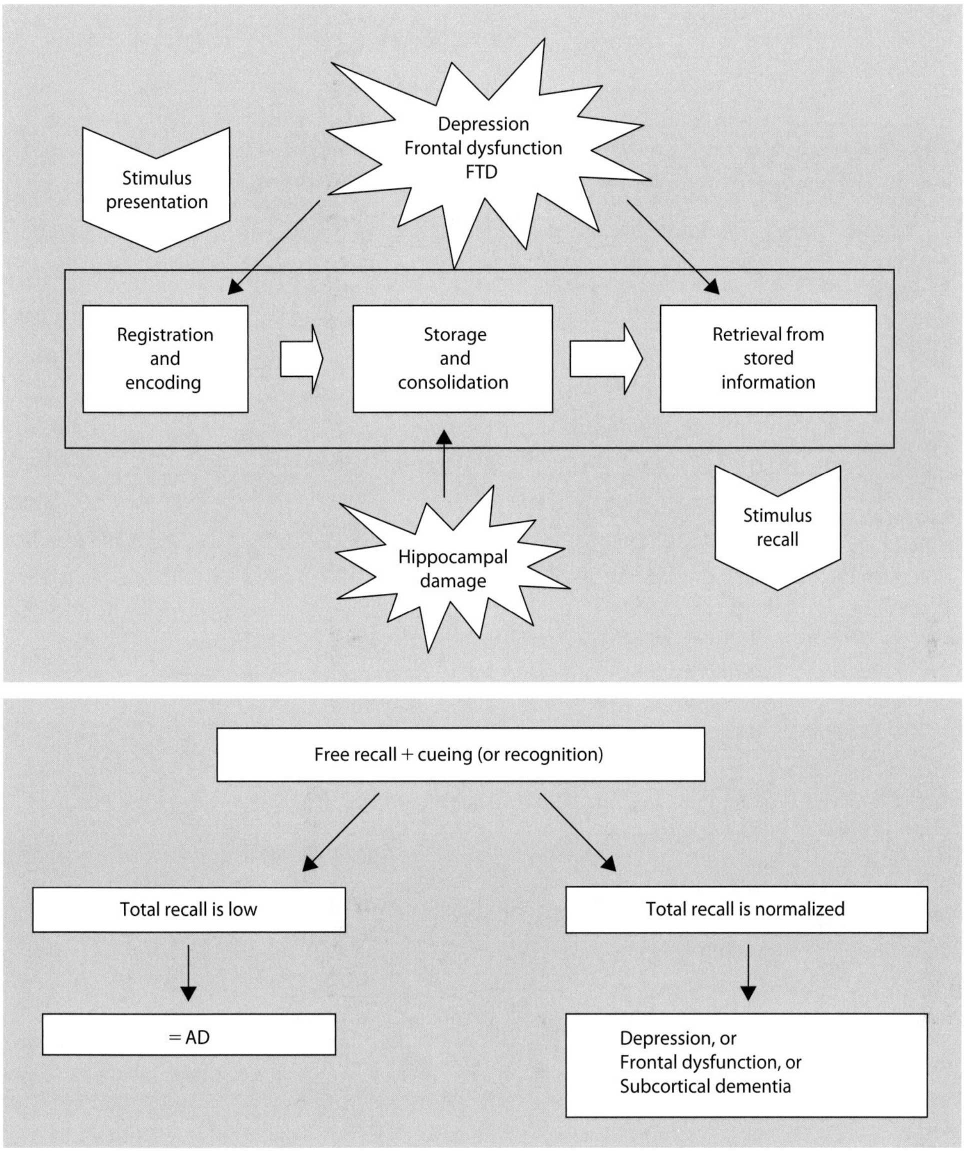

Fig. 1. Principle of examination of long-term memory. FTD = Frontotemporal dementia.

reactive serum syphilis serology, suspicion of other conditions (metastasis cancer, CNS infection, CNS vasculitis or Creutzfeldt-Jakob disease) [22].

The importance of biomarkers in clinical practice has increased in recent years. There are three markers in the CSF that have been studied: the Aβ42 protein, the total tau (t-tau) and the phospho-tau (p-tau). These markers reflect the pathogenic processes of amyloid aggregation and hyperphosphorylation of the tau protein. Some studies have demonstrated correlations between biomarkers and neuropathology

Table 1. Causes of dementia

Cortical degenerative dementia without motor sign
AD
Frontotemporal dementia: frontal dementia; progressive non fluent aphasia, semantic dementia, FTD
Other focal neurodegenerative syndromes: progressive visuospatial impairment, progressive apraxia
Subcortical degenerative dementia with motor sign
Parkinson disease with dementia
Progressive supranuclear palsy
Huntington's disease
Cortico-subcortical degenerative dementia with motor sign
Dementia with Lewy bodies
Corticobasal degeneration
Multiple system atrophy
Vascular dementia
Multi-infarct dementia
Strategic infarct-related dementia
Binswanger's encephalopathy
CADASIL (hereditary vascular dementia)
Cerebral amyloid angiopathy
White matter lesions
Mixed dementia
Infectious dementia
Syphilis
Whipple disease
HIV-related dementia
Virus encephalitis (herpes encephalitis)
Progressive multifocal leukoencephalopathy
Subacute sclerosing panencephalitis
Prion protein disease
Creutzfeldt Jakob; Kuru; fatal familial insomnia; Gerstmann-Sträussler-Scheinker disease
Dementia associated with toxic causes
Lead, mercury, aluminium, solvents
Carbon monoxide and anoxy
Radiotherapy, chemotherapy
Alcohol
Marchiafava-Bignami disease
Dementia associated with autoimmune disease or inflammatory disorders
Multiple sclerosis
Systemic lupus erythematosus
Behçet's disease
Sjögren's syndrome
Vasculitis with or without systemic involvement
Sarcoidosis
Metabolic dementia
Wilson disease
B_{12} deficiency, thyroid disease, parathyroid disease

[23], as well as hippocampal atrophy [24]. In AD, the concentration of Ab42 in cerebrospinal fluid is low and t-tau is high compared with those in healthy controls. Several recent studies have addressed the value of cerebrospinal fluid biomarkers in identifying early AD. A combination of CSF t-tau and Aβ42 at baseline yielded a sensitivity of 95% and a specificity of 83% for detection of incipient AD in patients with MCI [25]. The relative risk of progression to AD was substantially increased in MCI patients who had pathological concentrations of t-tau and Aβ42 at baseline [25].

Other studies have also shown that biomarkers may have a predictive value in recognizing MCI patients who will convert into AD [26, 27].

Neuroimaging

For many years, the use of the CT and MRI in the evaluation of AD has been restricted to excluding neurosurgical lesions, such as brain tumors or subdural hematomas, or to investigate evidence of cerebrovascular lesions (cerebral infarcts, white matter lesions) that may account for vascular dementia. However, modern neuroimaging extends beyond this traditional role of excluding other conditions. New MRI techniques can investigate both the structural and functional abnormalities that are specific to AD [28]. While neuroimaging can show cerebral atrophy, visualized as enlarged ventricles and cortical sulci, the overlap with normal aging and other dementias is too large to have any diagnostic value in clinical practice.

However, MRI can assess the presence of medial temporal lobe atrophy, which reflects the degenerative changes in the hippocampus and entorhinal cortex caused by the disease. The volume of the hippocampus, measured by MRI, is significantly reduced in AD compared to control subjects [28].

With the development of more efficient techniques for recognizing predementia conditions, it is expected that the importance of neuroimaging in the clinical practice will increase, both for the early diagnosis and follow-up of the patient.

Familial Genetic Mutations

Three autosomal dominant mutations that cause AD have been identified on chromosomes 21 (amyloid precursor protein), 14 (presenilin 1), and 1 (presenilin 2) [29]. The presence of a proband with genetic testing for one of these mutations can be considered strongly supportive for the diagnosis of AD [8].

Differential Diagnosis

Other medical, neurological, or psychiatric disorders which could account for the impairment in memory and related symptoms must be investigated.

Other neurodegenerative dementia (table 1) could be questioned particularly in following cases:

- Early behavioral disturbances, particularly social misconduct and eating changes, could be indicative of frontotemporal dementia.
- Early extrapyramidal signs, early visual hallucinations, early visuospatial and attentional impairment, REM sleep behavioural disorders and symptom fluctuation could be caused by Lewy body dementia.
- Vascular dementia is implicated by the presence of vascular lesions in neuroimaging and a sudden onset with focal neurological signs.
- Early language disorders could be caused by progressive nonfluent aphasia (hesitant, effortful speech and agrammatism), semantic dementia (progressive loss of knowledge about words and objects), or logopenic progressive aphasia (progressive decrease in speech output with anomia).
- Onset presenting with higher-order visuospatial dysfunction, Balint syndrome (ocular apraxia, optic ataxia, simultanagnosia) could be indicative of progressive posterior cortical atrophy.

Acknowledgements

Leonardo Cruz de Souza was supported by a grant from Association France Alzheimer.

References

1 Nestor PJ, Scheltens P, Hodges JR: Advances in the early detection of Alzheimer's disease. Nat Med 2004;10(suppl):S34–S41.

2 De Leon MJ, Mosconi L, Blennow K, DeSanti S, Zinkowski R, Mehta PD, Pratico D, Tsui W, Saint Louis LA, Sobanska L, Brys M, Li Y, Rich K, Rinne J, Rusinek H: Imaging and CSF studies in the preclinical diagnosis of Alzheimer's disease. Ann N Y Acad Sci 2007;1097:114–145.

3 Cummings JL: Alzheimer's disease. N Engl J Med 2004;351:56–67.

4 Hodges JR: Alzheimer's centennial legacy: origins, landmarks and the current status of knowledge concerning cognitive aspects. Brain 2006;129:2811–2822.

5 Braak H, Braak E: Neuropathological staging of Alzheimer-related changes. Acta Neuropathol (Berl) 1991;82:239–259.

6 Godbolt AK, Cipolotti L, Watt H, Fox NC, Janssen JC, Rossor MN: The natural history of Alzheimer disease: a longitudinal presymptomatic and symptomatic study of a familial cohort. Arch Neurol 2004;61:1743–1748.

7 Grober E, Buschke H, Crystal H, Bang S, Dresner R: Screening for dementia by memory testing. Neurology 1988;38:900–903.

8 Dubois B, Feldman HH, Jacova C, Dekosky ST, Barberger-Gateau P, Cummings J, Delacourte A, Galasko D, Gauthier S, Jicha G, Meguro K, O'brien J, Pasquier F, Robert P, Rossor M, Salloway S, Stern Y, Visser PJ, Scheltens P: Research criteria for the diagnosis of Alzheimer's disease: revising the NINCDS-ADRDA criteria. Lancet Neurol 2007;6: 734–746.

9 Tounsi H, Deweer B, Ergis AM, Van der Linden M, Pillon B, Michon A, Dubois B: Sensitivity to semantic cuing: an index of episodic memory dysfunction in early Alzheimer disease. Alzheimer Dis Assoc Disord 1999;13:38–46.

10 Dubois B, Slachevsky A, Litvan I, Pillon B: The FAB: a Frontal Assessment Battery at bedside. Neurology 2000;55:1621–1626.

11 Celone KA, Calhoun VD, Dickerson BC, Atri A, Chua EF, Miller SL, DePeau K, Rentz DM, Selkoe DJ, Blacker D, Albert MS, Sperling RA: Alterations in memory networks in mild cognitive impairment and Alzheimer's disease: an independent component analysis. J Neurosci 2006;26:10222–10231.

12 Morris JC: The Clinical Dementia Rating (CDR): current version and scoring rules. Neurology 1993;43:2412–2414.

13 Folstein MF, Folstein SE, McHugh PR: 'Mini Mental State'. A practical method for grading the cognitive state of patients for the clinician. J Psychiatr Res 1975;12:189–198.

14 Burback D, Molnar FJ, St. John P, Man-Son-Hing M: Key methodological features of randomized controlled trials of Alzheimer disease therapy: minimal clinically important difference, sample size and trial design. Dement Geriatr Cogn Disord 1999; 10:534–540.

15 Sarazin M, Stern Y, Berr C, Riba A, Albert M, Brandt J, Dubois B: Neuropsychological predictors of dependency in patients with Alzheimer disease. Neurology 2005;64:1027–1031.

16 Starkstein SE, Jorge R, Mizrahi R, Robinson RG: A prospective longitudinal study of apathy in Alzheimer's disease. J Neurol Neurosurg Psychiatry 2006;77:8–11.

17 Scarmeas N, Albert M, Brandt J, Blacker D, Hadjigeorgiou G, Papadimitriou A, Dubois B, Sarazin M, Wegesin D, Marder K, Bell K, Honig L, Stern Y: Motor signs predict poor outcomes in Alzheimer disease. Neurology 2005;64:1696–1703.

18 McKhann G, Drachman D, Folstein M, Katzman R, Price D, Stadlan EM: Clinical diagnosis of Alzheimer's disease: report of the NINCDS-ADRDA Work Group under the Auspices of Department of Health and Human Services Task Force on Alzheimer's disease. Neurology 1984;34:939–944.

19 Blacker D, Albert MS, Bassett SS, Go RC, Harrell LE, Folstein MF: Reliability and validity of NINCDS-ADRDA criteria for Alzheimer's disease. The National Institute of Mental Health Genetics Initiative. Arch Neurol 1994;51:1198–1204.

20 Pillon B, Deweer B, Agid Y, Dubois B: Explicit memory in Alzheimer's, Huntington's, and Parkinson's diseases. Arch Neurol 1993;50:374–379.

21 Sarazin M, Berr C, De Rotrou J, Fabrigoule C, Pasquier F, Legrain S, Michel B, Puel M, Volteau M, Touchon J, Verny M, Dubois B: Amnestic syndrome of the medial temporal type identifies prodromal AD: a longitudinal study. Neurology 2007;69:1859–1867.

22 Sampson EL, Warren JD, Rossor MN: Young onset dementia. Postgrad Med J 2004;80:125–139.

23 Buerger K, Ewers M, Pirttila T, Zinkowski R, Alafuzoff I, Teipel SJ, DeBernardis J, Kerkman D, McCulloch C, Soininen H, Hampel H: CSF phosphorylated tau protein correlates with neocortical neurofibrillary pathology in Alzheimer's disease. Brain 2006;129:3035–3041.

24 Hampel H, Bürger K, Prussner JC, Zinkowski R, DeBernardis J, Kerkman D, Leinsinger G, Evans AC, Davies P, Möller HJ, Teipel SJ: Correlation of cerebrospinal fluid levels of tau protein phosphorylated at threonine 231 with rates of hippocampal atrophy in Alzheimer Disease. Arch Neurol 2005;62:770–773.

25 Hansson O, Zetterberg H, Buchhave P, Londos E, Blennow K, Minthon L: Association between CSF biomarkers and incipient Alzheimer's disease in patients with mild cognitive impairment: a follow-up study. Lancet Neurol 2006;5:228–234.

26 Ewers M, Buerger K, Teipel SJ, Scheltens P, Schröder J, Zinkowski RP, Bouwman FH, Schönknecht P, Schoonenboom NS, Andreasen N, Wallin A, DeBernardis JF, Kerkman DJ, Heindl B, Blennow K, Hampel H: Multicenter assessment of CSF-phosphorylated tau for the prediction of conversion of MCI. Neurology 2007;69:2205–2212.

27 Li G, Sokal I, Quinn JF, Leverenz JB, Brodey M, Schellenberg GD, Kaye JA, Raskind MA, Zhang J, Peskind ER, Montine TJ: CSF tau/Abeta42 ratio for increased risk of mild cognitive impairment: a follow-up study. Neurology 2007;69:631–639.

28 Lehéricy S, Marjanska M, Mesrob L, Sarazin M, Kinkingnehun S: Magnetic resonance imaging of Alzheimer's disease. Eur Radiol 2007;17:347–362.

29 Mattson MP: Pathways towards and away from Alzheimer's disease. Nature 2004;430:631–639.

Marie Sarazin, MD, PhD
Fédération des Maladies du Système Nerveux
Research and Resource Memory Centre, Pavillon Paul Castaigne
Hôpital de la Salpêtrière, 47 Bd de l'Hôpital, FR–75013 Paris (France)
Tel. +33 1 42 16 19 86, Fax +33 1 42 16 27 39, E-Mail marie.sarazin@psl.aphp.fr

Giannakopoulos P, Hof PR (eds): Dementia in Clinical Practice.
Front Neurol Neurosci. Basel, Karger, 2009, vol 24, pp 12–19

The Concept of Mild Cognitive Impairment: Relevance and Limits in Clinical Practice

Agnès Michon

Division of Geriatric Psychiatry, Department of Psychiatry, University Hospitals of Geneva, Chêne-Bourg, Geneva, Switzerland

Abstract

Subtle cognitive impairments without dementia are common in the elderly population and numerous nosological entities have been proposed for their classification. The concept of mild cognitive impairment has become increasingly popular both in clinical practice and in research. It has been developed to describe a transitional zone between the cognitive changes of normal aging and early Alzheimer's disease or other forms of dementia. Its interest lies mainly in early identification of individuals who might be at risk of developing rapid cognitive decline. But the further one tends towards the early detection, the greater is the risk to lose in specificity. A number of other factors such as depression, metabolic or nutritional disorders, medication use, may cause cognitive dysfunctions and are reversible. The concept of mild cognitive impairment arouses a debate about its heterogeneity, limits, and relevance in clinical practice and research.

The clinical diagnosis of dementia is currently supported by specific criteria requiring the presence of a memory disorder associated with impairment in at last one additional cognitive domain, severe enough to interfere with social function or activities of daily living [1]. The main concern in defining these dementia criteria was to differentiate people with dementia from those with cognitive changes associated with physiological aging. However, most of pathological processes underlying dementia have a progressive course and early symptoms occur before clinically overt dementia. Therefore, the main difficulty resides in the early identification of patients with degenerative or vascular disease or who have a high risk of showing a subsequent cognitive decline and ultimately convert to dementia. Many patients evaluated mainly for a memory cognitive complaint are neither cognitively intact nor are they impaired enough to be classified as having very mild dementia. This transitional stage which is characterized by subtle cognitive deficits (primarily but not exclusively memory deficit) is referred to as mild cognitive impairment (MCI).

This grey area raises several questions and debates about its real relevance in daily clinical practice: how to characterize this condition, what are its determinants and what is its temporal evolution?

Evolution of Concepts

The problem of the wide spectrum of cognitive deficits between normal ageing and dementia has been approached by two different ways: first, by studying the general population complaining about cognitive changes irrespective of the etiology or the potential evolution, secondly by focusing on the early features of Alzheimer's disease (AD) and other dementia.

Various concepts close to MCI started to appear in the literature more than 40 years ago [for review, see 2]. The first to be proposed was the benign senescent forgetfulness defined by Kral in 1962 [3] in opposition to the 'malignant' senescent forgetfulness. It was centered on the memory impairment including an inability to recall minor detail, forgetting of remote as opposed to recent events and awareness of memory problems. Other conceptualizations have followed Kral's benign senescent forgetfulness. Crook et al. [4] in 1986 developed the notion of age-associated memory impairment (AAMI) referring to memory complaints of gradual onset in elderly people substantiated by a decrease of at least one standard deviation on a formal memory test. A problem with AAMI was that the performance was compared with young adults' norms, so that AAMI became highly prevalent in the elderly population. The late-life forgetfulness concept [5] modified the Crooks criteria by adding an upper age limit, requiring standardized self-report memory questionnaires and using results from a battery of tests based on age-matched norms. In 1994, in the concept of ageing-associated cognitive decline [6], age standardization, taking cohort effect into account and a broader focus integrating other functions than memory such as attention and concentration, thinking, language and visuospatial abilities was proposed. A similar concept is the age-related cognitive decline described concomitantly in the DSM-IV [1]. It refers to an objective decline in cognitive functioning due to a physiological process of ageing and is defined as a complaint of difficulties in recalling names, appointments, or in problem solving which cannot be related to a specific mental problem or a neurological disorder. Strikingly, the age-related cognitive decline definition specified neither a specific assessment procedure nor a reference group. All of these early concepts considered mild cognitive changes associated with ageing as intrinsic to the ageing process. Alternatively, it has been supposed that mild cognitive changes could be caused by an underlying disease and could be harbingers of disease. Within this theoretical framework, the International Classification of Disease (ICD-10) [7] included the concept of mild cognitive disorder that refers to disorders of memory and learning or concentration often accompanied by mental fatigue. These disorders must be shown by formal neuropsychological testing and attributable to cerebral disease or damage, or physical disease known to cause dysfunction, excluding dementia amnesic syndrome brain injury or postencephalitis syndrome. The mild neurocognitive disorder in the DSM-IV [1] was a conceptually similar diagnosis which includes not only memory problems but also executive functions, linguistic and perceptual-motor abilities. Both early disease and age-related problems were included in the category cognitive impairment no dementia proposed in the Canadian Study of Health and Aging [8] that encompasses many disorders from circumscribed memory impairment to chronic alcohol and drug use, psychiatric illness, mental retardation, and vascular pathologies which did not meet the criteria for dementia. Cognitive impairment no dementia was a broad and poorly delineated diagnostic category which concerned elderly individuals with cognitive impairment in several cognitive domains that often but not (consistently) progress to dementia [9].

At the same time and in parallel to these qualitative approaches, two main scales have been proposed using scales classifying people from cognitively normal to dementia. The Global Deterioration Scale [10] or The Clinical Dementia Rating Score [11] permits to identify memory impairment or other changes as predementia syndromes. MCI corresponds to stage 2 or 3 on the Global Deterioration Scale, and the 0.5 score on the Clinical Dementia Rating is designated as 'questionable dementia' (0 = normal and 1 = dementia).

Mild Cognitive Impairment

The concept of MCI was proposed by the Mayo Clinic group [12] to fill the gap between normal and dementia-type pathological ageing, and assumes that a cognitive continuum exists between normality and dementing disorders such as AD. The construct has been proposed to designate an early but abnormal state of cognitive impairment and has come to be recognized as a pathological condition and as a diagnostic entity, i.e. not a manifestation of normal ageing [13]. It is not generally thought to be a direct consequence of a systemic disease, but may be a significant risk factor for dementia, in particular AD. The original criteria (table 1) focused on the presence of memory problems and memory disorders characterizing MCI as a stage of memory impairment beyond aging but in which other cognitive domains were preserved and daily functions remained largely intact [14, 15]. In 1999 [12], these criteria were clarified: the absence of impaired cognitive function in a domain other than memory was required, memory tests claimed 1.5 standard deviation below normative values. This construct was essentially believed to be a clinical description of persons who were destined to develop AD [12]. In fact, most of the subsequent literature on MCI has focused on individuals who meet these criteria [16, 17].

One main problem of these criteria was their unilateral focus on memory deficit that contrasts with the frequent observation of nonmemory deficits among patients

Table 1. MCI initial criteria [12]

Memory complaint preferably corroborated by an informant
Objective memory impairment for age and education
Largely normal general cognitive functions
Essentially intact activities of daily living
Not demented

with cognitive complaints. Taking into account that not all forms of MCI progress to AD and therefore that other presentations of cognitive impairment needed to be considered, the Current Concepts in MCI Conference [15] proposed to distinguish three subtypes of MCI: (1) amnestic MCI, with only memory impairment, which will usually progress to AD; (2) multiple-domain slightly impaired MCI, with slight deficits in many cognitive domains without requiring memory deficit, which may progress to AD or other forms of dementia, and (3) MCI single nonmemory domain, with a single deficit in a cognitive domain other than memory, which may, according to the affected domain, progress to non-Alzheimer-type dementia such as frontotemporal dementia or primary progressive aphasia.

Some authors such as Dubois and Albert [18] argue that 'amnestic MCI' and 'multiple-domain slightly impaired MCI' are in fact AD in a presymptomatic stage so that these two classifications can also be called 'MCI of the Alzheimer type' or 'prodromal AD'. They propose diagnostic criteria for 'prodromal AD' including memory complaint, progressive onset, normal or mildly impaired complex activities of daily living, evidence of objective memory disorder based on a memory test showing the specificity of amnestic syndrome of the 'hippocampal type' (very poor free recall despite adequate encoding, limited effect of cueing on recall or impaired recognition, numerous intrusions), persistence of memory changes at a subsequent assessment, absence of the fully developed syndrome of dementia and exclusion of other disorders that may cause MCI, with adequate tests, including neuroimaging and biomarkers.

An etiology-oriented diagnostic procedure for MCI has recently been discussed by the Working Group of the European Consortium on AD [19]. A classification has been proposed for use in clinical practice, corresponding to the subtypes usually encountered in outpatient care: cognitive disorders corresponding to neurodegenerative disease (pre-AD MCI, Lewy body dementia or frontotemporal dementia, and more rarely focal atrophy); cognitive disorders corresponding to vascular lesions (vascular predementia MCI, mixed dementia); dysphoric or dysthymic disorder (anxious or depressive syndrome). The diagnostic procedure proposed would make it possible to identify patients at high risk for progression to dementia with additional tests (such as analysis of CSF and neuroimaging) required for determining the underlying cause.

Determinants and Course of Mild Cognitive Impairment

The prevalence of MCI and its subtypes varies greatly, ranging from 3% to around 13% of people older than 65 years, depending on the criteria used and population studied (general or memory clinic cohort) [20]. Epidemiological studies suggest that the progression of MCI is heterogeneous and may be reversible (some studies have shown that up to 40% of the subjects with MCI will improve at follow-up) [20–22]. In the case of an amnestic MCI of a presumed degenerative etiology, the most likely outcome will be AD. The rate of progression to AD is 10–15% per year [23]. Several neuropsychological markers of conversion to dementia have been proposed for the amnestic form of MCI including episodic memory tasks (verbal and nonverbal at different retrieval conditions such as free recall, recognition and immediate versus delayed recall [for review, see 24]), semantic memory and visuospatial functions [25]. From a structural viewpoint, the association between the rate of hippocampal atrophy and amnestic MCI conversion is now well established [26]. Modern neuropathological studies have shown that mesial temporal lobe atrophy starts in the context of normal brain aging and clearly precedes the development of the first neuropsychological deficits. It is thus not surprising that several studies attempted to identify a functional marker of MCI progression to AD. After a period of positive data, there is now increasing skepticism about the validity of functional neuroimaging as a tool in the early diagnosis of AD. This is partly due to the great variability of suggested associations at least in studies at resting state and to the marked heterogeneity of the MCI. Most importantly, in the absence of activation paradigms, numerous studies revealed metabolic and regional blood flow differences with unclear biological significance. As a consequence, to date none of these measures have a high predictive value in an individual case [26].

Limits

The main criticism towards the MCI construct is that it is only descriptive, difficult to operationalize and probably not a biologically early diagnosis. Most of these definitions use insufficiently detailed criteria. This may lead to variability in application of the criteria as well as in results [27]. Objective cognitive impairment must be diagnosed on the basis of evidence, but neuropsychological aspects of the classification are poorly defined and no limits have been proposed. The evaluation method varies greatly from one study to another, depending on the type of population analyzed, and on the objectives of the study. 'All-purpose' consensus-based or reference batteries currently do not exist [19]. There is a lack of clarity between the boundaries of MCI and so-called normal people and MCI and dementia. In particular, the distinction between amnestic MCI and early AD is very subtle and the demarcation is difficult to draw [18, 27]. Some authors argue that clinical judgment is not sufficient and propose neuropsychological instruments [28]. Furthermore, the criteria corresponding to absence of repercussions on daily life may be too restrictive, insofar as cognitive disorders may have slight repercussions on complex day-to-day activities. Adequate tools for its evaluation need to be specified. The psychological and behavioral symptoms should also be taken into account and should not systematically be the exclusion criteria for the diagnosis. Patients may have depressive symptoms related to cognitive impairment or to the underlying process. Dierckx et al. [28] propose to incorporate depressive symptoms in the diagnostic procedure of Petersen [12], assuming that elderly depression with concomitant cognitive problems can be seen as MCI.

The concept of MCI is also criticized as a syndromal description and as an unstable condition since many subjects do not worsen over time and may revert to normal cognitive abilities. Thus, for some authors [27], MCI is considered as unable to characterize subjects who share a prognosis or who may benefit from treatment and as not a clinically useful concept. Furthermore, the label of predementia stage does subjects, who revert to normal, harm.

Most importantly, the notion of a biologically early diagnosis has been profoundly changed during the last years after the identification of functional compensation phenomena in MCI. Most early studies in this field focused on functions subserved by the hippocampal formation which is known to be compromised very early in the course of the degenerative process [for review see 29]. Recent studies demonstrated that MCI cases are able to compensate the initial functional deficits by activating alternative cortical circuits in order to achieve correct execution of cognitive tasks [30]. In respect of pharmacological findings and in contrast to that originally expected, two studies correlated levels of hippocampal choline acetyltransferase (ChAT) activity with the extent of AD lesions in control, MCI, and AD cases. MCI subjects presented with increased hippocampal ChAT activity [31, 32]. This elevation was no longer present in mild AD cases, which were not different from controls. Severe AD cases showed markedly depleted hippocampal ChAT levels. These observations suggest that the development of compensatory mechanisms takes place early in normal brain aging and may at least partly account for the differences observed between MCI and controls but also between MCI converters and nonconverters.

Utility in Clinical Practice

Despite its ambiguities, the concept of MCI remains useful in highlighting the importance of considering the cognitive complaints in elderly people. Its utility concerns the detection of patients at high risk of progressing to AD or dementia disorders and to propose a follow-up to them in order to improve early diagnosis and early treatment. It is clear that not all will progress to dementia, and that MCI is an interim diagnosis. As such, clinicians should pay attention to not stigmatize these patients and not take this diagnosis lightly [33]. It is important to assess the various conditions potentially associated with memory or cognitive complaints, such as anxiety or depression, side effects of drugs, particularly anticholinergic agents, alcohol abuse, hypothyroidism, nutritional deficiency, or sleep apnea. After identifying the 'MCI syndrome' on the basis of memory complaint, decline in cognitive functioning relative to previous abilities (referring to a questionnaire or a battery of cognitive tests repeated at 6-month intervals) and cognitive deficits evidenced by clinical evaluation without major repercussions on daily life, the second step is to review which MCI subtype (amnestic or nonamnestic, single or multiple domain) and which underlying etiopathogenic subtype (neurodegenerative disease, vascular lesions, dysthymic disorders) are involved [19].

Effective treatments of MCI have not been demonstrated as yet. Several clinical trials for amnestic MCI with anticholinesterase inhibitors have been unsuccessful. This apparent lack of sustained benefit might be explained by different ways: by the compensatory upregulation of central cholinergic activity [32], by the lack of sensitivity of the cognitive outcome or by the heterogeneity of patients. Vascular risk factor should be treated more carefully, and lifestyle changes such as diet, physical and leisure activities can be counseled [34].

References

1 American Psychiatric Association: Diagnostic and Statistical Manual of Mental Disorders DSM-IV. American Psychiatric Association, Washington, 1994.

2 Davis HS, Rockwood K: Conceptualization of mild cognitive impairment: a review. Int J Geriatr Psychiatry 2004;19:313–319.

3 Kral VA. Senescent forgetfulness: benign and malignant. J Can Med Assoc 1962;86:257–260.

4 Crook T, Bartus RT, Ferris SH, Whitehouse P, Cohen GD, Gershon S: Age-associated memory impairment: proposed diagnostic criteria and measures of clinical change – Report of a National Institute of Mental Health work group. Dev Neuropsychol 1986; 2:261–276.

5 Blackford RC, La Rue A: Criteria for diagnosing age associated memory impairment: proposed improvements from the field. Dev Neuropsychol 1989;5:295–306.

6 Levy R: Aging-associated cognitive decline. Working Party of the International Psychogeriatric Association in collaboration with the World Health Organization. Int Psychogeriatr 1994;6:63–68.

7 World Health Organization: The ICD-10 Classification of Mental and Behavioural Disorders. Diagnostic Criteria for Research World Health Organization. Geneva, World Health Organization, 1993.

8 Graham JE, Rockwood K, Beattie EL, McDowell I, Eastwood R, Gauthier S: Standardization of the diagnosis of dementia in the Canadian Study of Health and Aging. Neuroepidemiology 1996;15:246–256.

9 Tuokko H, Frerichs RJ, Graham JE, Rockwood K, Kristjansson B, Fisk J, Bergman H, Kozma A, McDowell I: Five year follow-up of cognitive impairment with no dementia. Arch Neurol 2003;60:577–582.

10 Reisberg B, Ferris SH, DeLeon MJ, Crook T: The global deterioration scale for assessment of primary degenerative dementia. Am J Psychiatry 1982;139: 1136–1139.

11 Hughes CP, Berg L, Danziger WL, Coben LA, Martin RL: A new clinical scale for the staging of dementia. Br J Psychiatry 1982;140:566–572.

12 Petersen RC, Smith GE, Waring SC: Mild cognitive impairment: clinical characterization and outcome. Arch Neurol 1999;56:303–308.

13 Petersen RC: Mild cognitive impairment as a diagnostic entity. J Int Med 2004;256:183–194.

14 Petersen RC, Smith GE, Waring SC, Ivnik RJ, Kokmen E, Tangelos EG: Aging, memory, and mild cognitive impairment. Int Psychogeriatr 1997;9:65–69.

15 Petersen RC, Doody R, Kurz A, Mohs RC, Morris JC, Rabins PV, Ritchie K, Rossor M, Thal L, Winblad B: Current concepts in mild cognitive impairment. Arch Neurol 2001;58:1985–1992.
16 Gauthier S, Reisberg B, Zaudig M, Petersen RC, Ritchie K, Broich K, Belleville S, Brodaty H, Bennett D, Chertkow H, Cummings JL, de Leon M, Feldman H, Ganguli M, Hampel H, Scheltens P, Tierney MC, Whitehouse P, Winblad B, International Psychogeriatric Association Expert Conference on mild cognitive impairment: Mild cognitive impairment. Lancet 2006;367:1262–1270.
17 Ritchie K, Touchon J: Mild cognitive impairment: conceptual basis and current nosological status. Lancet 2000;355:225–228.
18 Dubois B, Albert M: Amnestic MCI or prodromal Alzheimer's disease? Lancet Neurol 2004;3:246–248.
19 Portet F, Ousset PJ, Visser PJ, Frisoni GB, Nobili F, Scheltens P, Vellas B, Touchon J, the MCI Working Group of the European Consortium of Alzheimer's disease (EADC): Mild cognitive impairment (MCI) in medical practice: a critical review of the concept and new diagnostic procedure. Report of the MCI Working Group of the European Consortium of Alzheimer's Disease. J Neurol Neurosurg Psychiatry 2006;77:714–718.
20 DeCarli C: Mild cognitive impairment: prevalence, prognosis, aetiology and treatment. Lancet Neurol 2003;2:15–21.
21 Ganguli M, Dodge HH, Shen C, DeKosky ST: Mild cognitive impairment, amnestic type: an epidemiological study. Neurology 2004;63:115–121.
22 Ritchie K. Artero S, Touchon J: Classification criteria for mild cognitive impairment: a population-based validation study. Neurology 2001;56:37–42.
23 Petersen RC: Mild cognitive Impairment: current research and clinical implications. Semin Neurol 2007;27:22–31.
24 Chetelat G, Eustache F, Viader F, De La Sayette V, Pélerin A, Mézenge F, Hannequin D, Dupuy B, Baron JC, Desgranges B: FDG-PET measurement is more accurate than neuroposychological assessments to predict global cognitive deterioration in patients with mild cognitive impairment. Neurocase 2005;11:14–25.
25 Artero S, Tierney MC, Touchon J, Ritchie K: Prediction of transition from mild cognitive impairment to senile dementia: a prospective, longitudinal study. Acta Psychiatr Scand 2003;107:390–393.
26 Wolf H, Jelic V, Gertz HJ, Nordberg A, Julin P, Wahlund LO: A critical discussion of the role of neuroimaging in mild cognitive impairment. Acta Neurol Scand Suppl 2003;179:52–76.
27 Visser PJ, Brodaty H: MCI is not a clinically useful concept. Int Psychogeriatr 2006;18:402–409.
28 Dierckx E, Engelborghs S, De Raedt R, De Deyn PP, Ponjaert-Kristoffersen I: Mild cognitive impairment: what's in a name? Gerontology 2007;53:28–35.
29 Missonnier P, Gold G, Fazio-Costa L, Michel JP, Mulligan R, Michon A, Ibáñez V, Giannakopoulos P: Early event-related potential changes during working memory activation predict rapid decline in mild cognitive impairment. J Gerontol A Biol Sci Med Sci 2005;60:660–666.
30 Rosano C, Aizenstein HJ, Cochran JL, Saxton JA, De Kosky ST, Newman AB, Kuller LH, Lopez OL, Carter CS: Event-related functional magnetic resonance imaging investigation of executive control in very old individuals with mild cognitive impairment. Biol Psychiatry 2005;57:761–767.
31 Ikonomovic MD, Mufson EJ, Wuu J, Cochran EJ, Bennett DA, DeKosky ST: Cholinergic plasticity in hippocampus of individuals with mild cognitive impairment: correlation with Alzheimer's neuropathology. J Alzheimer Dis 2002;5:39–48.
32 DeKosky ST, Ikonomovic MD, Styren SD, Beckett L, Wisniewski S, Bennett DA, Cochran EJ, Kordower JH, Mufson EJ: Upregulation of choline acetyltransferase activity in hippocampus and frontal cortex of elderly subjects with mild cognitive impairment. Ann Neurol 2002;51:145–155.
33 Petersen RC, Knopman DS: MCI is a clinically useful concept. Int Psychogeriatr 2006;18:394–402.
34 Gauthier S: Is mild cognitive impairment (MCI) a clinically useful concept? Commentary. Int Psychogeriatr 2006;18:409.

Dr. Agnès Michon
Psychiatry Department, Division of Geriatric Psychiatry
University Hospitals of Geneva (HUG)
2, chemin du Petit-Bel-Air, CH–1225 Chêne-Bourg, Geneva (Switzerland)
Tel. +41 22 305 50 09, Fax +41 22 305 50 44, E-Mail agnes.michon@hcuge.ch

Giannakopoulos P, Hof PR (eds): Dementia in Clinical Practice.
Front Neurol Neurosci. Basel, Karger, 2009, vol 24, pp 20–29

Pathological Substrates of Cognitive Decline in Alzheimer's Disease

Panteleimon Giannakopoulos[a,c] · Enikö Kövari[a] · Gabriel Gold[b] · Armin von Gunten[c] · Patrick R. Hof[d,e] · Constantin Bouras[a,d]

Departments of [a]Psychiatry and [b]Geriatrics, University of Geneva School of Medicine, Chêne-Bourg, Geneva, [c]Division of Old Age Psychiatry, University of Lausanne School of Medicine, Lausanne, Switzerland; Departments of [d]Neuroscience and [e]Geriatrics and Adult Development, Mount Sinai School of Medicine, New York, N.Y., USA

Abstract

The progressive development of Alzheimer's disease (AD)-related lesions such as neurofibrillary tangles, amyloid deposits and synaptic loss within the cerebral cortex is a main event of brain aging. Recent neuropathologic studies strongly suggested that the clinical diagnosis of dementia depends more on the severity and topography of pathologic changes than on the presence of a qualitative marker. However, several methodological problems such as selection biases, case-control design, density-based measures, and masking effects of concomitant pathologies should be taken into account when interpreting these data. In last years, the use of stereologic counting permitted to define reliably the cognitive impact of AD lesions in the human brain. Unlike fibrillar amyloid deposits that are poorly or not related to the dementia severity, the use of this method documented that total neurofibrillary tangles and neuron numbers in the CA1 field are the best correlates of cognitive deterioration in brain aging. Loss of dendritic spines in neocortical but not hippocampal areas has a modest but independent contribution to dementia. In contrast, the importance of early dendritic and axonal tau-related pathologic changes such as neuropil threads remains doubtful. Despite these progresses, neuronal pathology and synaptic loss in cases with pure AD pathology cannot explain more than 50% of clinical severity. The present review discusses the complex structure/function relationships in brain aging and AD within the theoretical framework of the functional neuropathology of brain aging.

Alzheimer's Disease-Type Lesions in Brain Aging: Introductory Remarks

The progressive development of Alzheimer's disease (AD)-related pathology in the cerebral cortex constitutes a major event that occurs in the human brain as a function of age. Yet, the exact cognitive repercussions of these changes remain controversial. Since Tomlinson's first observations [1], several neuropathological studies have confirmed that neurofibrillary tangles (NFT), and amyloid deposits may be present in the hippocampal formation and restricted parties of the mesial temporal lobe in most elderly people with either very mild memory impairment or even in the absence of cognitive deterioration [2, 3]. Furthermore, amyloid deposits are also found even within neocortical association areas in intellectually preserved elderly individuals [4, 5]. Altogether, these data imply that the diagnosis of AD is not related to the presence or absence of a specific pathological hallmark but depends instead on the severity and distribution of AD type lesions in the brain (fig. 1). Contrasting with this theoretical position, certain authors have stressed the importance of qualitative differences between brain aging and AD such as the presence of Aβ40-immunoreactive reticular amyloid deposits and PHF-positive senile plaques or the substantial neuronal loss in the CA1 field, yet the validity of these markers is still not widely accepted [6]. In clinically overt dementia, a substantial NFT formation within adjacent components of the medial and inferior aspects of the temporal cortex and later on in other neocortical association areas was reported, whereas there were only weak correlations between fibrillar amyloid deposits and cognitive status in demented cases [7, 8]. The relationship between the pattern and densities of NFT and amyloid deposits in brain aging and in AD has led to the development of neuropathologic staging models of AD. In 1991, Braak and Braak developed an NFT-based model to differentiate initial, intermediate and advanced stages of AD [9]. Nine years after the first description of the NFT staging system, Braak's group described a new amyloid-based model. This newer model describes four phases in the evolution of amyloid Aβ deposition within the medial temporal lobe, which are significantly correlated with the Braak NFT-based stages [10].

Tau-related neuronal pathology is not confined to NFT. It also includes pretangles defined as non fibrillar accumulations of tau, and end-stage extracellular NFT that were usually taken into account in clinicopathological correlations [11]. Besides these perikarya-related types of neuronal pathology, neuropil threads (NT) in dendrites and axons contain paired helical filaments composed of hyperphosphorylated tau. Clinically, this neuritic pathology is of considerable interest as it is thought to account for 85–90% of cortical tau pathology in normal brain aging and early AD [12]. Some investigators have postulated that NFT in the soma and NT in the processes of neurons are formed simultaneously [13], while others argue that NT formation precedes NFT formation in most neurons [14]. In this context, an increase in NT has been reported in cases with mild cognitive impairment followed by a substantial decrease in severe AD. In contrast to the well-established impact of NFT in cognition, the clinical significance of NT remains controversial [14].

Several studies have shown that in addition to NFT and amyloid deposits, AD is characterized by selective neuronal loss [15], severe and early loss of synapses [16], and synaptic pathology [17]. Early immunocytochemical studies indicated an average 30–45% decrease in presynaptic terminal density in the AD neocortex [17]. The contribution of Terry et al. [18] first implied that severity of AD is more robustly

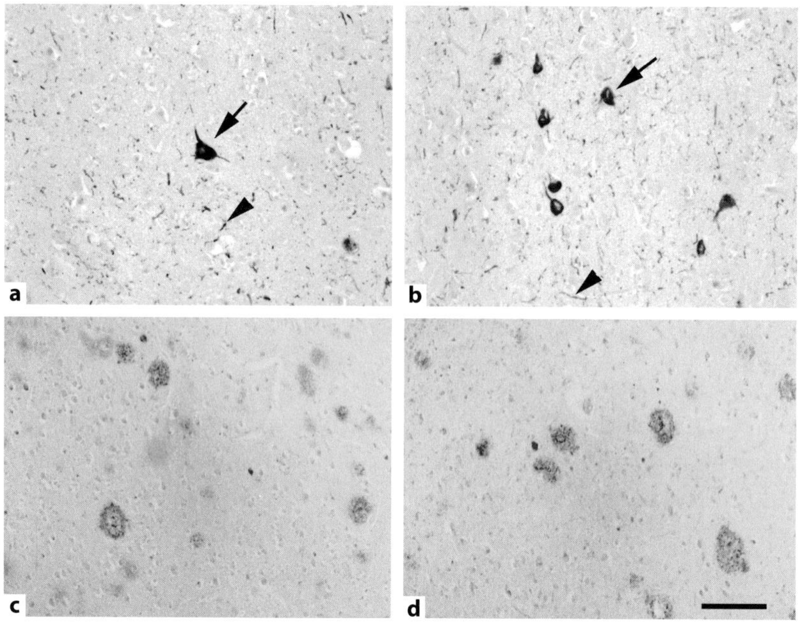

Fig. 1. Representative examples of Alzheimer-type lesions in normal aging (**a, c**) and AD (**b, d**). **a, b** NFT (arrows) and threads (arrowheads); **c, d** Senile plaques in the entorhinal cortex. Immunohistochemistry with anti-tau (**a, b**) and anti-amyloid (**c, d**) antibodies. Scale bar: 100 μm (**a, b**); 200 μm (**c, d**).

related to synapse loss than amyloid plaque, tangle densities, degree of neuronal loss, or extent of cortical gliosis. In particular, they postulated that synaptophysin immunoreactivity, a widely used presynaptic marker, decreases in the prefrontal cortex of AD cases, explaining about 70% of the global psychometric test variability [18]. Recent reports revealed synaptophysin reduction in NFT-containing neurons in the hippocampus and association cortices in mild cognitive impairment and early AD, pointing to the relationship between NFT formation and loss of presynaptic markers [19].

In contrast to presynaptic markers, AD changes in postsynaptic structures have been rarely studied. Spines are dynamic structures that are the proposed site of synaptic plasticity underlying learning and memory [20]. Because of the distance of dendritic extent from the soma, dendritic spines may be particularly vulnerable to incipient degenerative processes that disrupt intracellular signaling and synaptic functions. Spinophilin, a synaptic protein implicated in spine formation and synaptic transmission, displays a remarkably distinct localization to the heads of majority of dendritic spines in all brain regions examined, although the concentration per spine is regionally and locally variable. Spinophilin immunoreactivity has been shown to be intense in the majority of dendritic spines of rat hippocampus [21]. It is present in about 93% of the dendritic spines in rhesus monkey hippocampus, but sparsely distributed in other portions of the dendrites, making it an excellent marker for quantitative assessment of spine numbers [22].

Methodological difficulties should be also considered when interpreting these observations. From a strictly technical point of view, the first period of clinicopathological correlations in AD were based on lesion densities that are subject to major sampling biases. For instance, estimates of synaptic loss relied upon density measures and nonsystematic sampling based on two unwarranted assumptions, namely that the size of the region under analysis remains constant across diagnostic groups and that synaptic size does not change [23]. In addition, most studies concerned limited autopsy series and used an 'all or nothing' approach without calculating the relative contribution of each type of lesions in cognitive decline. Finally, although multivariate analyses have been classically used to control for the effect of demographic variables, apolipoprotein E genotype, or number of affected areas, only rare contributions have attempted to control for the interdependence of AD pathologic hallmarks in the aging brain [24, 25]. The present review summarizes recent clinicopathological data related to AD pathology in elderly cohorts without vascular pathology and discusses their relevance in the context of the long-lasting efforts to define the pathological substrates of cognitive deterioration in the elderly.

Pathological Determinants of Cognition in Cases with Alzheimer-Type Lesions: Neurofibrillary Tangles, Amyloid Deposits or Neuronal Loss?

In the field of pure AD, the positive association between clinical severity estimated by the Clinical Dementia Rating (CDR) scores and neuropathologic staging was highly significant for both NFT and Aβ protein deposition classification [26]. However, the strength of the relationship was greater for NFT-based Braak staging. In a univariate model, it accounted for 26.5% of the variability in clinical severity as measured by the CDR, whereas Aβ protein deposition staging accounted for 13.0% and age for 4.4%. In a multivariate analysis including the two neuropathologic classifications and age, the model explained 30.1% of the variability in CDR scores. NFT and age together accounted for 27.2% and the addition of Aβ protein staging to the model could only explain an extra 2.9% of the clinical variability.

Although this is a key finding, such studies have the weakness of leaving a large part of the clinical variability unexplained. This may be in part due to methodological issues related to the relative coarseness of the scales that were used (5 levels of cognition for the CDR and 4 or 6 stages for the pathological classifications). Subsequent studies using the 30-point MMSE scale and rigorous stereological assessment of the number of NFTs and amyloid volume [27] showed that a very high proportion of the variability in MMSE scores was explained by NFT and neuronal counts in the CA1 field (83 and 85.4%), entorhinal cortex (87.8 and 83.7%) and area 9 (87 and 79%) (fig. 2). Importantly, total amyloid volume in all of the

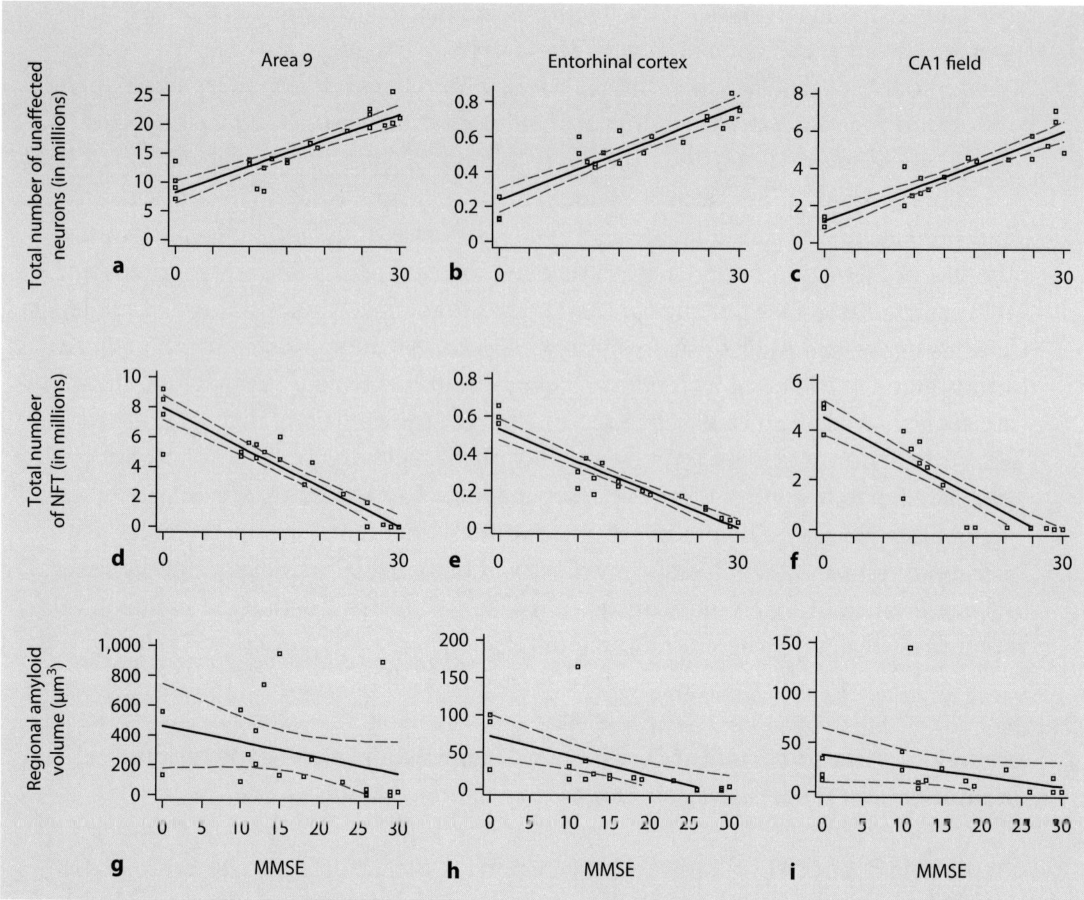

Fig. 2. Total number of unaffected neurons (**a–c**), NFT (**d–f**), and amyloid volume (**g–i**) in area 9 (**a, d, g**), entorhinal cortex (**b, e, h**) and CA1 field (**c, f, i**) as a function of dementia severity measured by the MMSE score. Note the strong relationship between MMSE scores and total number of unaffected neurons as well as NFT numbers in studied areas. This was not the case for total amyloid volume. Reproduced with permission from Giannakopoulos et al. [27].

areas studied was not significantly related to MMSE score in any of the above multivariate models.

Supporting the marginal cognitive impact of fibrillar amyloid deposits, these results indicate that the reported cognitive correlates of amyloid load in univariate analyses mainly reflect its correlation with NFT [25]. Most importantly, they indicate that total NFT counts and neuron numbers in area 9 and the hippocampus are highly predictive of cognitive status. Contrasting with the more modest performance of NFT-Braak staging [26], NFT numbers in the entorhinal cortex or area 9 could predict more than 87% of the variability in MMSE scores. The stereologic assessment of neuronal loss but also NFT numbers in neocortical areas remains of course a time-consuming process not easily compatible with routine neuropathologic work. However, based on these observations which show an excellent correlation between total NFT numbers in the entorhinal cortex and MMSE scores (compared to the semiquantitative assessment proposed by Braak), one could recommend the systematic assessment of total NFT numbers in the entorhinal cortex and CA1 field as a unique pathologic marker of AD progression.

One main conceptual problem that remained concerns the limited age range of the sample used in most clinicopathological studies with a clear underrepresentation of oldest-old individuals. The extensive analysis of total NFT and neuron numbers in the entorhinal cortex and CA1 field in an independent series of 34 individuals encompassing the whole spectrum of old age and CDR scores revealed that cognitive variability is only partly explained using a pure 'lesional' model of reference [28]. Questionable dementia was associated with a 1.9% neuronal loss in the entorhinal cortex and 26% in the CA1 field. Importantly, even in cases with overt clinical signs of dementia, more than 60% of pyramidal neurons in the CA1 field were still present further supporting the notion of the persistence of a substantial neuronal reserve in this particular area even in late stages of the degenerative process [29]. Estimates of both neuronal loss and NFT numbers in the CA1 field seems to be the best correlate of cognitive decline explaining 44% of the CDR variability. These results imply that in contrast to our observations in younger cohorts, NFT or neuron numbers in the hippocampal formation still explain less than 50% of the variability in CDR scores when the whole spectrum of brain aging is taken into account.

Neuropil Threads Do Not Affect Cognition in Brain Aging

Despite their predominance in the initial stages of AD neurodegeneration, the temporal relationship between the formation of NT and progressive invasion of the hippocampus by AD lesions is unclear. In terms of their evolution in dementia, a recent study of NT length in the hippocampus and entorhinal cortex of 19 very old individuals with various degrees of cognitive decline showed that this length increases in both the hippocampus and frontal cortex in mildly demented cases but showed a marked decrease in the CDR score of 3 cases [30]. This observation parallels that of Mitchell et al. [14] who reported an increase in NT in cases with mild cognitive impairment with a subsequent decrease in cases with moderate to severe AD and postulated that their toxic effect in hosting dendrites results in degeneration and resorption. This hypothesis has also been supported by Sassin et al. [31] who provided a morphological description of this phenomenon in NFT-containing neurons of the nucleus basalis of Meynert. Alternatively, the decrease in NT length may reflect the fact that the constant gain related to the addition of newly produced tau in the early stages of the degenerative process may cease in severe cases as a consequence of NT disconnection from the cell body.

In terms of cognitive impact, early contributions yielded positive data but were based on case-control designs and density measures in vulnerable cortical areas [32, 33]. Thal et al. [10] also found that the proportion of cases with NT in hippocampal subdivisions is higher among mildly demented cases, supporting a possible deleterious role of NT in cognition. More recently, Mitchell et al. [14] failed to identify a relationship between NT burden in entorhinal cortex and memory dysfunction in cases with various degrees of cognitive decline. The first stereologic data in this field revealed that the cognitive impact of NT on the hippocampal formation is limited to the CA1 field and remains strictly mediated by their relationship to NFT. Consistent with that previously reported with respect to NFT [28], total NT lengths were not related to CDR scores in the entorhinal cortex. Univariate models revealed a modest contribution of CA1 NT in dementia severity, yet this association did not persist when NFT was considered as an additional dependent variable in multivariate models. This finding challenges the usefulness of assessing systematically NT burden at least in routine neuropathologic settings.

Dendritic Spine Loss in Neocortex Independently Predicts Dementia

Using both a global neuropsychological measure (MMSE) and a dementia severity scale (CDR), a recent study in 16 elderly individuals revealed that the loss of dendritic spines in CA1 field and area 9 has a strong negative impact on cognition [34]. This overall observation agrees with several earlier and recent contributions stressing the role of synapses in AD cognitive decline [16–19]. In particular, the univariate models showed that total numbers of spinophilin-immunoreactive puncta in the CA1 field and area 9 might explain more than 20 and 60% of MMSE variability. Unusually high percentages of explained variability (18% for CA1 field and 42% for area 9) were also obtained when the CDR score was used as a dependent variable.

However, the strong predictive value of spinophilin-immunoreactive puncta counts in CA1 field did not persist when adjusting for Braak NFT staging in multivariate models, indicating that the cognitive repercussion of dendritic spine loss in this area is strictly mediated by the global NFT burden. Our quantitative data also confirmed this observation showing that, in terms of clinicopathologic correlations, total NFT number is the main marker to consider in this area. Importantly, they also show that the local depletion of pyramidal neurons and loss of spinophilin-immunoreactive puncta are independent phenomena which contribute separately to the cognitive decline. A different pattern was present in area 9 where spinophilin-immunoreactive puncta numbers remained significantly associated with cognitive measures after controlling for Braak NFT staging and explained an additional 17.5% of MMSE variability and 15% of CDR variability. These results imply that neocortical but not hippocampal dendritic spine loss may be an independent parameter to explore in AD clinicopathologic correlations.

Conclusions

The identification of relevant neuropathologic hallmarks of cognitive deterioration should not mask the relative dissociation between clinical expression and traditionally assessed AD pathology. In cases with pure AD pathology, more than 50% of CDR variability cannot be explained by NFT, amyloid deposits and neuronal loss in the hippocampal formation [28]. An attractive scenario for these cases would be that the development of synaptic loss may be more closely related to cognitive impairment than NFT formation and neuronal loss. However, the independent effect of synaptic loss (at least with respect to postsynaptic elements) seems to be rather modest and mostly confined to neocortical areas. Alternatively, neuropathologic parameters other than lesions may determine cognitive performance. In this respect, the state of brain microvessels is an attractive candidate since it is closely related to the adaptive capacities of the human brain. A recent stereologic analysis revealed that the mean microvessel diameters in entorhinal cortex and, to a lesser degree the CA1, were independent predictors of cognitive status in very old individuals supporting further a direct role of microvascular integrity in cognition [35]. Decreased microvessel diameters may lead to impaired microcirculation within the hippocampal formation and thus prevent adaptive responses to local changes in metabolic demands. Moving away from the logic of a unique relationship between lesion development and loss of function, these new data suggest that structural parameters that influence brain function such as the state of cortical microvasculature may be an additional determinant of cognition.

Acknowledgements

We thank Drs C.B. Rivara, A.B. Rocher, F.R. Herrmann and T. Bussière for their participation in some of the studies discussed in this review. B. Wicinski, P. Lovero and M. Demiri provided excellent technical help. This work was supported by NIH grants AG02219 and AG05138 (P.R.H.) and the Jérôme Tissières Foundation (P.G.).

References

1 Tomlinson BE, Blessed G, Roth M: Observations on the brains of non-demented old people. J Neurol Sci 1968;7:331–356.

2 Bennett DA, Schneider JA, Arvanitakis Z, Kelly JF, Aggarwal NT, Shah RC, Wilson RS: Neuropathology of older persons without cognitive impairment from two community-based studies. Neurology 2006;66: 1837–1844.

3 Knopman DS, Parisi JE, Salviati A, Floriach-Robert M, Boeve BF, Ivnik RJ, Smith GE, Dickson DW, Johnson KA, Petersen LE, McDonald WC, Braak H, Petersen RC: Neuropathology of cognitively normal elderly. J Neuropathol Exp Neurol 2003;62:1087–1095.

4 Hof PR, Bierer LM, Perl DP, Delacourte A, Buée L, Bouras C, Morrison JH: Evidence for early vulnerability of the medial and inferior aspects of the temporal lobe in an 82 year old patient with preclinical signs of dementia: regional and laminar distribution of neurofibrillary tangles and senile plaques. Arch Neurol 1992;49:946–953.

5 Masliah E, Mallory M, Hansen L, DeTeresa R, Terry RD: Quantitative synaptic alterations in the human neocortex during normal aging. Neurology 1993;43:192–197.

6 Dickson DW: Neuropathological diagnosis of Alzheimer's disease: a perspective from longitudinal clinicopathological studies. Neurobiol Aging 1997;18:S21–S26.

7 Berg L, McKeel DW Jr, Miller JP, Storandt M, Rubin EH, Morris JC, Baty J, Coats M, Norton J, Goate AM, Price JL, Gearing M, Mirra SS, Saunders AM: Clinicopathologic studies in cognitively healthy aging and Alzheimer's disease: relation of histologic markers to dementia severity, age, sex, and apolipoprotein e genotype. Arch Neurol 1998;55:326–335.

8 Riley KP, Snowdon DA, Desrosiers MF, Markesbery WR: Early life linguistic ability, late life cognitive function, and neuropathology: findings from the nun study. Neurobiol Aging 2005;26:341–347.

9 Braak H, Braak E: Neuropathological stageing of Alzheimer-related changes. Acta Neuropathol (Berl) 1991;82:239–259.

10 Thal DR, Rüb U, Schultz C, Sassin I, Ghebremedhin E, Del Tredici K, Braak E, Braak H: Sequence of Abeta-protein deposition in the human medial temporal lobe. J Neuropathol Exp Neurol 2000;59:733–748.

11 Braak E, Braak H, Mandelkow EM: A sequence of cytoskeleton changes related to the formation of neurofibrillary tangles and neuropil threads. Acta Neuropathol (Berl) 1994;87:554–567.

12 Mitchell TW, Nissanov J, Han LY, Mufson EJ, Schneider JA, Cochran EJ, Bennett DA, Lee VM, Trojanowski JQ, Arnold SE: Novel method to quantify neuropil threads in brains from elders with or without cognitive impairment. J Histochem Cytochem 2000;48:1627–1638.

13 Togo T, Akiyama H, Iseki E, Uchikado H, Kondo H, Ikeda K, Tsuchiya K, de Silva R, Lees A, Kosaka K: Immunohistochemical study of tau accumulation in early stages of Alzheimer-type neurofibrillary lesions. Acta Neuropathol (Berl) 2004;107:504–508.

14 Mitchell TW, Mufson EJ, Schneider JA, Cochran EJ, Nissanov J, Han LY, Bienias JL, Lee VM, Trojanowski JQ, Bennett DA, Arnold SE: Parahippocampal tau pathology in healthy aging, mild cognitive impairment, and early Alzheimer's disease. Ann Neurol 2002;51:182–189.

15 Hof PR, Cox K, Morrison JH: Quantitative analysis of a vulnerable subset of pyramidal neurons in Alzheimer's disease. I. Superior frontal and inferior temporal cortex. J Comp Neurol 1990;301:44–54.

16 Scheff SW, Price DA, Schmitt FA, Mufson EJ: Hippocampal synaptic loss in early Alzheimer's disease and mild cognitive impairment. Neurobiol Aging 2006;27:1372–1384.

17 Masliah E, Terry RD, Alford M, DeTeresa R, Hansen LA: Cortical and subcortical patterns of synaptophysin-like immunoreactivity in Alzheimer's disease. Am J Pathol 1991;138:235–246.

18 Terry RD, Masliah E, Salmon DP, Butters N, DeTeresa R, Hill R, Hansen LA, Katzman R: Physical basis of cognitive alterations in Alzheimer's disease: synapse loss is the major correlate of cognitive impairment. Ann Neurol 1991;30:572–580.

19 Masliah E, Mallory M, Alford M, DeTeresa R, Hansen LA, McKeel DW Jr, Morris JC: Altered expression of synaptic proteins occurs early during progression of Alzheimer's disease. Neurology 2001;56:127–129.

20 Segal M: Dendritic spines: elementary structural units of neuronal plasticity. Prog Brain Res 2002;138:53–59.

21 Allen PB, Ouimet CC, Greengard P: Spinophilin, a novel protein phosphatase 1 binding protein localized to dendritic spines. Proc Natl Acad Sci USA 1997;94:9956–9961.

22 Hao J, Janssen WG, Tang Y, Roberts JA, McKay H, Lasley B, Allen PB, Greengard P, Rapp PR, Kordower JH, Hof PR, Morrison JH: Estrogen increases the number of spinophilin-immunoreactive spines in the hippocampus of young and aged female rhesus monkeys. J Comp Neurol 2003;465:540–550.

23 Wolf H, Jelic V, Gertz HJ, Nordberg A, Julin P, Wahlund LO: A critical discussion of the role of neuroimaging in mild cognitive impairment. Acta Neurol Scand Suppl 2003;179:52–76.

24 Bancher C, Jellinger K, Lassmann H, Fischer P, Leblhuber F: Correlations between mental state and quantitative neuropathology in the Vienna Longitudinal Study on Dementia. Eur Arch Psychiatry Clin Neurosci 1996;246:137–146.

25 Grober E, Dickson D, Sliwinski MJ, Buschke H, Katz M, Crystal H, Lipton RB: Memory and mental status correlates of modified Braak staging. Neurobiol Aging 1999;20:573–579.

26 Gold G, Kövari E, Corte G, Herrmann FR, Canuto A, Bussière T, Hof PR, Bouras C, Giannakopoulos P: Clinical validity of a beta-protein deposition staging in brain aging and Alzheimer disease. J Neuropathol Exp Neurol 2001;60:946–952.

27 Giannakopoulos P, Herrmann FR, Bussière T, Bouras C, Kövari E, Perl DP, Morrison JH, Gold G, Hof PR: Tangle and neuron numbers, but not amyloid load, predict cognitive status in Alzheimer's disease. Neurology 2003;60:1495–1500.

28 von Gunten A, Kövari E, Bussière T, Rivara CB, Gold G, Bouras C, Hof PR, Giannakopoulos P: Cognitive impact of neuronal pathology in the entorhinal cortex and CA1 field in Alzheimer's disease. Neurobiol Aging 2006;27:270–277.

29 Kril JJ, Patel S, Harding AJ, Halliday GM: Neuron loss from the hippocampus of Alzheimer's disease exceeds extracellular neurofibrillary tangle formation. Acta Neuropathol (Berl) 2002;103:370–376.
30 Giannakopoulos P, von Gunten A, Kövari E, Gold G, Herrmann FR, Hof PR, Bouras C: Stereological analysis of neuropil threads in the hippocampal formation: Relationships with Alzheimer's disease neuronal pathology and cognition. Neuropathol Appl Neurobiol 2007;33:334–343.
31 Sassin I, Schultz C, Thal DR, Rub U, Arai K, Braak E, Braak H: Evolution of Alzheimer's disease-related cytoskeletal changes in the basal nucleus of Meynert. Acta Neuropathol (Berl) 2000;100:259–269.
32 Markesbery WR, Wang HZ, Kowall NW, Kosik KS, McKee AC: Morphometric image analysis of neuropil threads in Alzheimer's disease. Neurobiol Aging 1993;14:303–307.
33 McKee AC, Kosik KS, Kowall NW: Neuritic pathology and dementia in Alzheimer's disease. Ann Neurol 1991;30:156–165.
34 Akram A, Christoffel D, Rocher AB, Bouras C, Kövari E, Perl DP, Morrison JH, Herrmann FR, Haroutunian V, Giannakopoulos P, Hof PR: Stereologic estimates of total spinophilin-immunoreactive spine number in area 9 and the ca1 field: relationship with the progression of Alzheimer's disease. Neurobiol Aging 2008;29:1296–1307.
35 Bouras C, Kövari E, Herrmann FR, Rivara CB, Bailey TL, von Gunten A, Hof PR, Giannakopoulos P: Stereologic analysis of microvascular morphology in the elderly: Alzheimer disease pathology and cognitive status. J Neuropathol Exp Neurol 2006;65: 235–244.

Prof. Panteleimon Giannakopoulos
Division of Geriatric Psychiatry, Department of Psychiatry
University of Geneva School of Medicine
2, chemin du Petit-Bel-Air
CH–1225 Chêne-Bourg, Geneva (Switzerland)
Tel. +41 22 305 5001, Fax +41 22 305 5044
E-Mail Panteleimon.Giannakopoulos@medecine.unige.ch

Giannakopoulos P, Hof PR (eds): Dementia in Clinical Practice.
Front Neurol Neurosci. Basel, Karger, 2009, vol 24, pp 30–38

Functional Imaging in Mild Cognitive Impairment and Early Alzheimer's Disease: Is It Pertinent?

Vicente Ibáñez[a] · Marie-Pierre Deiber[b]

[a]Neuroimaging Unit, Department of Psychiatry, University Hospitals of Geneva, Chêne-Bourg, Geneva, Switzerland; [b]INSERM Unit 877, Faculty of Medicine, Grenoble, France

Abstract

Neuroimaging techniques, namely positron emission tomography (PET), single photon emission computed tomography (SPECT), and magnetic resonance imaging (MRI) are increasingly used to study mild cognitive impairment (MCI) and its conversion to dementia, as well as early Alzheimer's disease (AD). Despite an important overlap of the various imaging parameter values between MCI, early AD and controls, some markers may help clinical diagnosis in individual patients. For example, the combination of significantly reduced hippocampal volume and brain hypometabolism in a MCI patient establishes the anatomical and functional features seen in dementia. In association with clinical information, the topographic localization of the hypometabolism will help to precise the type of dementia. Functional brain activation studies using functional MRI and PET are not used for clinical purpose, but they allow to determine the differences between control and pathological states and thus to characterize the functional abnormalities specific to the disease. Finally, the use of biomarkers of the neuropathological lesions constitutes the most promising tool to accurately diagnose MCI and early AD patients.

In his daily clinical practice, the physician has to identify those individuals presenting with some cognitive disturbance but with preserved abilities of daily living. These subclinical cognitive disorders can indeed represent the earliest stage of dementia and the diagnosis of mild cognitive impairment (MCI) may be proposed when fulfilling required criteria [1]. Whether the patients present with memory only impairment or other cognitive deficits, they are at risk to develop Alzheimer's disease (AD) or other type of dementia. However, not all of them will become demented and some can even improve their cognitive status [2]. Therefore, when diagnosing MCI both the clinician and the patient would like to also have a prognosis. Will the patient develop dementia, and if so, which type of dementia? In the absence of curative treatment for

AD, there is nevertheless a major interest to delay the conversion of MCI to AD or the evolution to more severe forms of the disease. Indeed, it has been demonstrated that for comparable life expectancy, delaying the onset of AD will result in a reduction of full-time care costs. Therefore MCI and early AD patients are becoming a potential drug target for new therapies based on neurobiological approaches. Although the brain energy demand is abnormally reduced in early AD, it is possible to induce cerebral activation and thus to increase the cerebral blood flow or glucose metabolism. This capacity of the brain to functionally respond at early stage of the disease makes a treatment to delay or prevent further deteriorations possible.

Two main concerns arise from the above. First, the patients who will evolve to dementia should be discriminated from those who will not. Second, the type of dementia to which each individual patient will evolve should be determined. In brief, it should be possible to better classify the MCI patients by detecting the pathological landmarks of the disease responsible for the degenerative cognitive impairment. Nevertheless, MCI prospective clinical cohort studies conducted to determine the prevalence of this syndrome have shown variable results extending between 5 and 24% [3, 4]. This variability has several reasons, but arbitrary chosen neuropsychological tests and lack of consistent specific diagnosis criteria are the main factors.

Data from neuropathological studies suggest that some MCI patients probably already present the pathological landmarks of AD [5]. Yet, the clinician will not consider the MCI patient as demented and the diagnosis of AD will be delayed until a full dementia syndrome installs. Indeed, MCI spectrum is large and can indicate, or not, a transitional phase between normal cognitive state and dementia. In many cases, the differences between MCI and early AD are likely to be very subtle. Therefore extended criteria are needed to improve both sensitivity and specificity of the diagnosis.

If cognition results from the dynamical coordination among specialized brain areas, the disruption of anatomical connectivity by vascular or degenerative lesions in dementia may result in some cognitive deficits. These lesions, as well as the resulting functional impairment, may be detected using appropriate neuroimaging techniques. Functional neuroimaging is currently rising great expectancy as a potential diagnosis tool for AD [6]. The relevant question is whether functional imaging in MCI and in early AD could detect the progressive dysfunction and the neuropathological changes leading to dementia. Ideally, neuroimaging data should provide proofs of the functional impairment as well as the topography, intensity and type of the lesions. Indeed, a definite detection of the pathological substrate could theoretically confirm the diagnosis of AD or of other type of dementia.

Because of the diversity of available imaging techniques, several approaches are possible, each one looking into particular aspects of the cerebral abnormalities causing the cognitive impairment. By measuring the gray matter volume, structural magnetic resonance imaging (MRI) allows to quantify the degree of brain atrophy caused by degenerative neuronal loss. MRI spectroscopy measures biochemical changes related to neuronal function by measuring various brain metabolites. The *N*-acetyl-aspartate, which marks the neuronal density, and the myoinositol, exploring glial activity, can be measured among others. Besides, functional neuroimaging using positron emission tomography (PET), single photon emission tomography (SPECT) or functional MRI, provides the opportunity to explore aspects of cognitive dysfunction and cerebral hypometabolism. Finally, the neuropathological lesions described in AD, namely the senile plaques (SP) and the neurofibrillary tangles (NFT), can theoretically be detected with appropriate PET or SPECT biomarkers.

However, to be useful to the diagnosis of MCI and early AD, the neuroimaging parameters should present two important aspects, namely a good sensitivity with a small interindividual variability of the data measured, and a good specificity with a full characterization of the dementia type.

Regarding sensitivity, the neuroimaging parameter measured in healthy individuals should be, as much as possible, normally distributed, so that abnormal values can be accurately detected in any individual patient. When there is a large variability of the measure, inherent to the technique or to the data analysis, neuroimaging studies will be useful to gain insight about particular aspects of the pathology under study but not to categorize each patient in clinical routine. Repeating the study over time within each individual can reduce the interindividual variability of the measure and help to assess the evolution of the disease, but becomes expensive.

Regarding specificity, the neuroimaging parameter should delineate a specific feature which characterizes the neurodegenerative disease to which the MCI patient will evolve. However, as will be discussed, while clinicians have to reach a decision for each individual, most dementia imaging studies based on cohorts of patients show considerable overlap of the measure between groups.

The measure of hippocampal volume with MRI is well standardized and relatively simple for the experienced physician. Moreover, semiautomatic or automatic analysis has been developed. Cerebral and hippocampal atrophy can occur several years before a patient develops AD and is also present in preclinical AD [7]. Structural MRI volumetric studies in MCI patients show that medial temporal atrophy is probably the best predictor of the evolution to AD [8, 9] (fig. 1). However, this anatomical feature is not specific to AD and can also be observed in other types of dementia. Moreover, it is not established whether an individual patient with decreased hippocampal volume will develop dementia or not. Although the values of hippocampal volume overlap considerably among groups, detecting a significantly reduced hippocampal volume in an individual MCI patient posits for the evolution to dementia. In other cortical regions, volume measurement is hampered by the difficulty to unequivocally delimit anatomical boundaries. Such limitation increases the interindividual variability of the measure and strongly reduces its utility for the diagnosis of dementia.

In AD, but also in frontotemporal dementia, MRI spectroscopy studies have evidenced a decrease of *N*-acetyl-aspartate and an increase of *myo*inositol as a result of reduced neuronal activity and glial proliferation [10]. In MCI patients the amount of

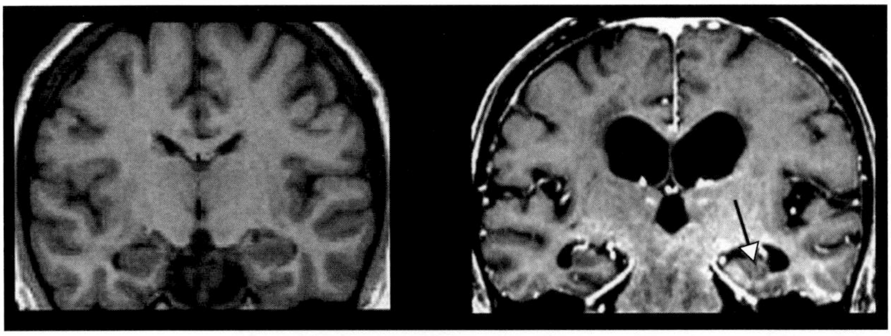

Fig. 1. Structural magnetic resonance images in a control and an early AD patient. Coronal slices show a reduction of hippocampal volume in AD (arrow).

metabolite changes are at midway between controls and AD patients [11]. These results need further validation before the technique may be used for clinical purpose.

Functional MRI and PET activation studies have not yet proved their utility in the diagnosis of MCI. Indeed, these techniques have inherent difficulties limiting their realization and the interpretation of the data. In terms of realization, limitations refer to the adaptation of the neuropsychological tests used for diagnosis to the experimental tasks of a neuroimaging protocol (e.g., patient lying still within an imaging device, control of actual engagement in the task). The other important limitation concerns the resolution of the signal amplitude. For example, the increase of oxyhemoglobin MRI signal in activated regions does not exceed 2 or 3%, rapidly showing ceiling effect. The increase of cerebral blood flow is larger with PET activation studies, but the restriction in radiation dose limits task repetition and thus statistical power in each individual. Functional MRI studies of MCI patients using memory tasks have given variable results, some of them suggesting that there could be a compensatory increase of hippocampal activation, while others have shown decreased activation in this structure as well as in other regions implicated in AD [12, 13]. Activation studies are therefore useful for research purpose but are not used for clinical diagnosis of MCI or dementia.

Brain glucose metabolism has been largely studied in AD and other types of dementia using ^{18}F-fluoro-2-deoxy-D-glucose (^{18}F-FDG) and PET. Interestingly, in early AD, the hippocampus has usually normal absolute glucose metabolism values in spite of the perceptible neuronal loss. High-energy demand from compensatory dendritic reactive outgrowth could contribute to maintain normal metabolic levels. But, with the evolution of the disease, there is a progressive decrease of glucose metabolism as shown by the negative correlation between age and hippocampus metabolism (fig. 2). On the other side, patients with clear dementia symptoms present cerebral hypometabolism within associative parietal areas, external temporal areas, precuneus, posterior cingulate cortex, the dorsolateral frontal cortex becoming affected with disease evolution [14]. This topography differs from frontotemporal dementia, in which the frontal lobes and anterior temporal lobes are preferentially concerned [15] (fig. 3). The

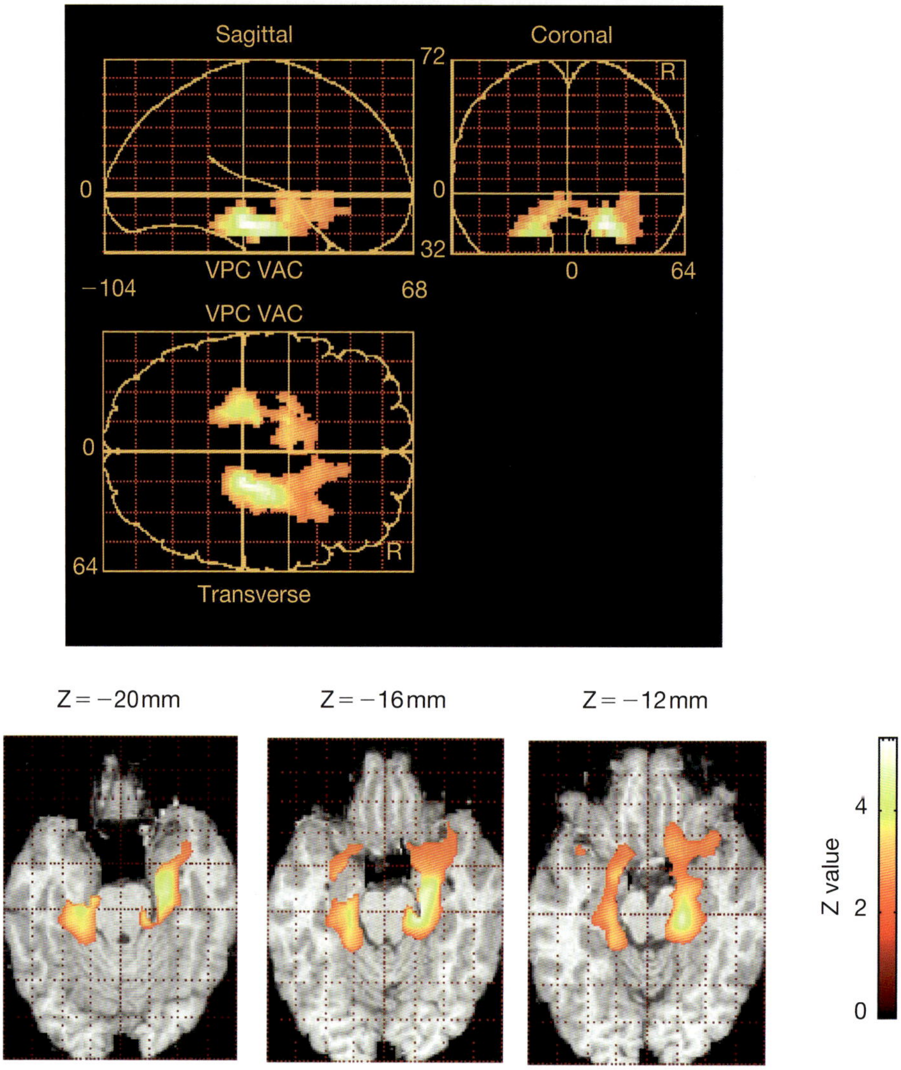

Fig. 2. Statistical parametric maps showing in the hippocampal formation of AD patients a significant negative correlation between PET glucose metabolism and age of diagnosis. Although absolute metabolism in the hippocampus is not significantly impaired at the beginning of the disease, it decreases with disease progression.

hypometabolism, which persists after correction for brain atrophy, does not depend on the degree of atrophy [16]. The high sensitivity and specificity of ^{18}F-FDG PET imaging to detect hypometabolism in confirmed AD patients prompted some authors to investigate subjects at risk. The ^{18}F-FDG results obtained from MCI cohort studies are encouraging, showing that as a group, the individuals at high risk to develop AD present a significant reduction of glucose metabolism compared to controls [17].

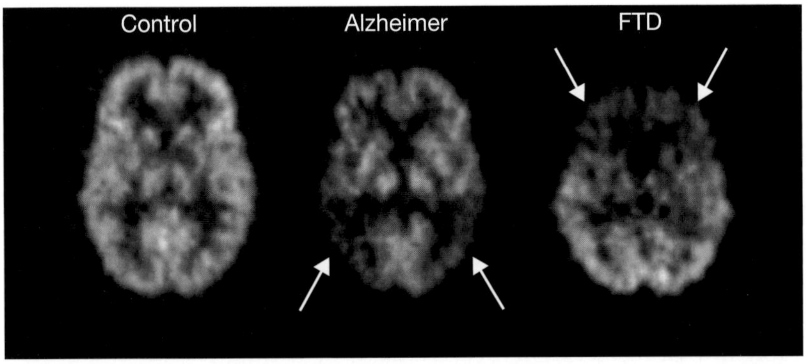

Fig. 3. PET imaging of glucose metabolism in a control subject, and two patients with AD and frontotemporal dementia. The topography of glucose hypometabolism clearly differs for the two patients. In AD the posterior part of the brain is more affected, while in frontotemporal dementia the frontal and anterior temporal lobes are preferentially concerned (arrows).

Therefore, although both sensitivity and specificity of the hypometabolism are lower for MCI than for AD diagnosis, reduced metabolism detected with ^{18}F-FDG PET in an MCI patient highly predicts the evolution to dementia [18].

PET molecular imaging using biomarkers constitutes a relatively recent aspect of neuroimaging studies in dementia. Its principle is to use labeled compounds that bind to characteristic AD lesions, namely the NFT and the SP. There are high expectations on the use of biomarkers since they could theoretically facilitate the early definite differential diagnosis between the dementia subtypes. Since a chapter of this book is devoted to the biomarkers in dementia, only an overview of some concepts useful for MCI diagnosis will be developed here. To be of real use for clinical diagnosis, the biomarkers should have a particularly high specificity for the neuropathological lesions, so that their binding pattern can differentiate the subtypes of dementia. Two main biomarkers are presently under investigation, the PIB component and the FDDNP [19]. The PIB binds preferentially to SP while the FDDNP binds to NFT, but with less specificity [20, 21]. There are few FDDNP studies in MCI patients since the discrimination power between controls and AD patients is lower for this compound than for the PIB. In contrast, PIB studies in MCI patients are developing, delineating two groups of patients: those with low PIB binding, similar to controls, and those with high PIB binding, similar to AD patients [22]. Moreover, a follow-up study suggests that MCI patients converting to AD have high level PIB binding [23]. However, it is not yet clear whether the use of PIB will improve the diagnosis and prognosis of MCI patients. Indeed, PIB binding has also been reported in controls without dementia or MCI syndrome [24]. Moreover, it is unclear why patients with frontotemporal dementia have increased PIB binding [25]. Two hypotheses can account for the findings on PIB, one related to the physiopathology and the other to the characteristics of PIB binding. First, in normal aging, cognitively normal individuals may present cerebral SP without developing AD. Second, PIB has been reported to bind not only to amyloid rich SP and to a lesser degree to NFT, but also to diffuse plaques as well as amyloid lesions in cerebrovascular amyloid angiopathy [26]. In addition, intriguingly, while SP extend and glucose metabolism decreases with disease severity, the amount of PIB binding does not seem to increase with evolution. On the other side of the spectrum, although less frequent, patients fulfilling the criteria for AD can present normal levels of PIB binding [27]. Another particular aspect of PIB is that in AD, it binds preferentially to the frontal cortex and striatum, although the SP are less abundant and the glucose metabolism is more preserved in these regions, at least at disease onset. It could be hypothesized that PIB additionally detects non-specific brain inflammation, or that the SP are not correlated to cognitive dysfunction in AD, in contrast to the NFT [28]. Another hypothesis could be that brain atrophy, more prominent in temporal and parietal associative regions, is responsible for the detection of a poorer PIB signal. Further studies are clearly needed to fully assess the significance of PIB binding in MCI, and the rate of false positive and false negative PIB scans. Furthermore, and since therapeutic research focuses on methods to stop the development of the abnormal tau protein, it would be essential to have a biomarker with high affinity for the NFT, the FDDNP compound not appearing as a good candidate because of its low specificity.

In parallel to the PET studies with biomarkers, efforts are made to visualize SP with MRI. In transgenic mice models developing cortical plaques, the MRI technique detects the plaques as areas of low signal [29]. While preliminary results are promising, more data must be acquired before applying the method to MCI and early AD patients.

Finally, indirect approaches focus on the detection of changes in serotonin or other neurotransmitter receptors as a result of cell death in hippocampus and entorhinal cortex. The density of serotonin receptors has been shown to increase in MCI as opposed to AD patients (upregulation), suggesting that compensatory mechanisms may exist at early stages of the degenerative process [30].

In conclusion, research efforts are needed to identify biomarkers with high specificity for each lesion type. With such biomarkers, the concept of MCI syndrome will be more restricted, since an accurate demonstration of the lesions would definitely posit the diagnosis of dementia.

References

1 Petersen RC, Smith GE, Waring SC, Ivnik RJ, Kokmen E, Tangelos EG: Aging, memory, and mild cognitive impairment. Int Psychogeriatr 1997;9 (suppl 1):65–69.

2 Busse A, Hensel A, Guhne U, Angermeyer MC, Riedel-Heller SG: Mild cognitive impairment: long-term course of four clinical subtypes. Neurology 2006;67:2176–2185.

3 Bennett DA, Wilson RS, Schneider JA, Evans DA, Beckett LA, Aggarwal NT, Barnes LL, Fox JH, Bach J: Natural history of mild cognitive impairment in older persons. Neurology 2002;59:198 205.

4 Hanninen T, Hallikainen M, Tuomainen S, Vanhanen M, Soininen H: Prevalence of mild cognitive impairment: a population-based study in elderly subjects. Acta Neurol Scand 2002;106:148–154.

5 Markesbery WR, Schmitt FA, Kryscio RJ, Davis DG, Smith CD, Wekstein DR: Neuropathologic substrate of mild cognitive impairment. Arch Neurol 2006; 63:38–46.

6 Dubois B, Feldman HH, Jacova C, Dekosky ST, Barberger-Gateau P, Cummings J, Delacourte A, Galasko D, Gauthier S, Jicha G, Meguro K, O'Brien J, Pasquier F, Robert P, Rossor M, Salloway S, Stern Y, Visser PJ, Scheltens P: Research criteria for the diagnosis of Alzheimer's disease: revising the NINCDS-ADRDA criteria. Lancet Neurol 2007;6: 734–746.

7 Fox NC, Warrington EK, Freeborough PA, Hartikainen P, Kennedy AM, Stevens JM, Rossor MN: Presymptomatic hippocampal atrophy in Alzheimer's disease. A longitudinal MRI study. Brain 1996;119:2001–2007.

8 DeCarli C, Frisoni GB, Clark CM, Harvey D, Grundman M, Petersen RC, Thal LJ, Jin S, Jack CR Jr, Scheltens P: Qualitative estimates of medial temporal atrophy as a predictor of progression from mild cognitive impairment to dementia. Arch Neurol 2007;64:108–115.

9 Jack CR Jr, Petersen RC, Xu YC, O'Brien PC, Smith GE, Ivnik RJ, Boeve BF, Waring SC, Tangalos EG, Kokmen E: Prediction of AD with MRI-based hippocampal volume in mild cognitive impairment. Neurology 1999;52:1397–1403.

10 Mihara M, Hattori N, Abe K, Sakoda S, Sawada T: Magnetic resonance spectroscopic study of Alzheimer's disease and frontotemporal dementia/ Pick complex. Neuroreport 2006;17:413–416.

11 Kantarci K, Jack CR Jr, Xu YC, Campeau NG, O'Brien PC, Smith GE, Ivnik RJ, Boeve BF, Kokmen E, Tangalos EG, Petersen RC: Regional metabolic patterns in mild cognitive impairment and Alzheimer's disease: A 1H MRS study. Neurology 2000; 55:210–217.

12 Johnson SC, Schmitz TW, Moritz CH, Meyerand ME, Rowley HA, Alexander AL, Hansen KW, Gleason CE, Carlsson CM, Ries ML, Asthana S, Chen K, Reiman EM, Alexander GE: Activation of brain regions vulnerable to Alzheimer's disease: the effect of mild cognitive impairment. Neurobiol Aging 2006;27:1604–1612.

13 Sperling R: Functional MRI studies of associative encoding in normal aging, mild cognitive impairment, and Alzheimer's disease. Ann N Y Acad Sci 2007;1097:146–155.

14 Friedland RP, Jagust WJ, Huesman RH, Koss E, Knittel B, Mathis CA, Ober BA, Mazoyer BM, Budinger TF: Regional cerebral glucose transport and utilization in Alzheimer's disease. Neurology 1989;39:1427–1434.

15 Herholz K: FDG PET and differential diagnosis of dementia. Alzheimer Dis Assoc Disord 1995;9:6–16.

16 Ibanez V, Pietrini P, Alexander GE, Furey ML, Teichberg D, Rajapakse JC, Rapoport SI, Schapiro MB, Horwitz B: Regional glucose metabolic abnormalities are not the result of atrophy in Alzheimer's disease. Neurology 1998;50:1585–1593.

17 Reiman EM, Caselli RJ, Yun LS, Chen K, Bandy D, Minoshima S, Thibodeau SN, Osborne D: Preclinical evidence of Alzheimer's disease in persons homozygous for the epsilon 4 allele for apolipoprotein E. N Engl J Med 1996;334:752–758.

18 Drzezga A, Grimmer T, Riemenschneider M, Lautenschlager N, Siebner H, Alexopoulos P, Minoshima S, Schwaiger M, Kurz A: Prediction of individual clinical outcome in MCI by means of genetic assessment and (18)F-FDG PET. J Nucl Med 2005;46:1625–1632.

19 Nordberg A: Amyloid imaging in Alzheimer's disease. Curr Opin Neurol 2007;20:398–402.

20 Klunk WE, Engler H, Nordberg A, Wang Y, Blomqvist G, Holt DP, Bergstrom M, Savitcheva I, Huang GF, Estrada S, Ausen B, Debnath ML, Barletta J, Price JC, Sandell J, Lopresti BJ, Wall A, Koivisto P, Antoni G, Mathis CA, Langstrom B: Imaging brain amyloid in Alzheimer's disease with Pittsburgh Compound-B. Ann Neurol 2004;55:306–319.

21 Small GW, Kepe V, Ercoli LM, Siddarth P, Bookheimer SY, Miller KJ, Lavretsky H, Burggren AC, Cole GM, Vinters HV, Thompson PM, Huang SC, Satyamurthy N, Phelps ME, Barrio JR: PET of brain amyloid and tau in mild cognitive impairment. N Engl J Med 2006;355:2652–2663.

22 Price JC, Klunk WE, Lopresti BJ, Lu X, Hoge JA, Ziolko SK, Holt DP, Meltzer CC, DeKosky ST, Mathis CA: Kinetic modeling of amyloid binding in humans using PET imaging and Pittsburgh Compound-B. J Cereb Blood Flow Metab 2005;25: 1528–1547.

23 Forsberg A, Engler H, Almkvist O, Blomquist G, Hagman G, Wall A, Ringheim A, Langstrom B, Nordberg A: PET imaging of amyloid deposition in patients with mild cognitive impairment. Neurobiol Aging 2007.

24 Mintun MA, Larossa GN, Sheline YI, Dence CS, Lee SY, Mach RH, Klunk WE, Mathis CA, DeKosky ST, Morris JC: [11C]PIB in a nondemented population: potential antecedent marker of Alzheimer disease. Neurology 2006;67:446–452.

25 Rabinovici GD, Furst AJ, O'Neil JP, Racine CA, Mormino EC, Baker SL, Chetty S, Patel P, Pagliaro TA, Klunk WE, Mathis CA, Rosen HJ, Miller BL, Jagust WJ: 11C-PIB PET imaging in Alzheimer disease and frontotemporal lobar degeneration. Neurology 2007;68:1205–1212.

26 Lockhart A, Lamb JR, Osredkar T, Sue LI, Joyce JN, Ye L, Libri V, Leppert D, Beach TG: PIB is a non-specific imaging marker of amyloid-beta (Abeta) peptide-related cerebral amyloidosis. Brain 2007; 130(Pt 10):2607–2615.
27 Edison P, Archer HA, Hinz R, Hammers A, Pavese N, Tai YF, Hotton G, Cutler D, Fox N, Kennedy A, Rossor M, Brooks DJ: Amyloid, hypometabolism, and cognition in Alzheimer disease: an [11C]PIB and [^{18}F]FDG PET study. Neurology 2007;68:501–508.
28 Giannakopoulos P, Herrmann FR, Bussiere T, Bouras C, Kovari E, Perl DP, Morrison JH, Gold G, Hof PR: Tangle and neuron numbers, but not amyloid load, predict cognitive status in Alzheimer's disease. Neurology 2003;60:1495–1500.
29 Jack C, Garwood M, Wengenack T, Borowski B, Curran G, Lin J, Adriany G, Grohn O, Grimm R, Poduslo J: In vivo visualization of Alzheimer's amyloid plaques by Magnetic Resonance Imaging in transgenic mice without a contrast agent. Magn Reson Med 2004;52:1263–1271.
30 Truchot L, Costes S, Zimmer L, Laurent B, Le Bars D, Thomas-Anterion C, Croisile B, Mercier B, Hermier M, Vighetto A, Krolak-Salmon P: Up-regulation of hippocampal serotonin metabolism in mild cognitive impairment. Neurology 2007; 69:1012–1017.

Vicente Ibáñez, MD, PhD
Neuroimaging Unit, Department of Psychiatry
2, chemin du Petit-Bel-Air
CH–1225 Chêne-Bourg, Geneva (Switzerland)
Tel. +41 22 305 5378, Fax +41 22 305 5375, E-Mail Vicente.Ibanez@hcuge.ch

Giannakopoulos P, Hof PR (eds): Dementia in Clinical Practice.
Front Neurol Neurosci. Basel, Karger, 2009, vol 24, pp 39–46

Electrophysiological Markers of Rapid Cognitive Decline in Mild Cognitive Impairment

Panteleimon Giannakopoulos[a,c] · Pascal Missonnier[a] · Enikö Kövari[a] · Gabriel Gold[b] · Agnès Michon[a]

Departments of [a]Psychiatry, and [b]Rehabilitation and Geriatrics, University Hospitals of Geneva, Chêne-Bourg, Geneva, [c]Division of Old Age Psychiatry, University Hospitals of Lausanne, Prilly, Switzerland

Abstract

Electroencephalography (EEG) is an easily accessible and low-cost modality that might prove to be a particularly powerful tool for the identification of subtle functional changes preceding structural or metabolic deficits in progressive mild cognitive impairment (PMCI). Most previous contributions in this field assessed quantitative EEG differences between healthy controls, MCI and Alzheimer's disease (AD) cases leading to contradictory data. In terms of MCI conversion to AD, certain longitudinal studies proposed various quantitative EEG parameters for an a priori distinction between PMCI and stable MCI. However, cross-sectional comparisons revealed a substantial overlap in these parameters between MCI patients and elderly controls. Methodological differences including variable clinical definition of MCI cases and substantial interindividual differences within the MCI group could partly explain these discrepancies. Most importantly, EEG measurements without cognitive demand in both cross-sectional and longitudinal designs have demonstrated limited sensitivity and generally do not produce significant group differences in spectral EEG parameters. Since the evolution of AD is characterized by the progressive loss of functional connectivity within neocortical association areas, event-modulated EEG dynamic analysis which makes it possible to investigate the functional activation of neocortical circuits may represent a more sensitive method to identify early alterations of neuronal networks predictive of AD development among MCI cases. The present review summarizes clinically significant results of EEG activation studies in this field and discusses future perspectives of research aiming to reach an early and individual prediction of cognitive decline in healthy elderly controls.

Predicting Cognitive Decline in Mild Cognitive Impairment: Evolution of the Concepts and New Challenges

The marked progress of pharmacological treatments as well as the first data supporting a future curative treatment based on vaccination against Aβ protein aroused increasing interest about the early identification of individuals at risk of developing Alzheimer's disease (AD). Although mild cognitive impairment (MCI) is considered a transitional stage in the pathogenesis of AD, not all MCI patients progress to clinically defined AD or decline at identical rates [for review, see 1]. In recent years, numerous neuroimaging studies addressed the issue of a biological predictive marker of further cognitive deterioration in MCI with conflicting data. Most of them were based on structural, metabolic or cerebral blood flow data in cross-sectional and longitudinal designs and focused on the progressive damage of hippocampal formation. Besides classical methodological limitations (number of cases, interindividual variability, epidemiological versus clinical sampling strategies), there are several conceptual problems that should be taken into account when attempting an early prediction of MCI conversion to dementia. First, MCI is a highly heterogeneous condition that includes three clinical subtypes (amnestic, multiple impaired cognitive domains, single nonmemory domain [2]). Second, the definition of conversion in terms of dichotomic outcome at a precise endpoint is not necessarily appropriate since patients who do not convert during the follow-up period include both patients who may convert later and patients who may never convert. Most importantly, the notion of early biological diagnosis has been profoundly changed during the last years after the identification of functional compensation phenomena in MCI. Most early studies in this field focused on functions subserved by the hippocampal formation that is known to be compromised very early in the course of the degenerative process [for review, see 3]. Recent studies demonstrated that MCI cases (but also high functioning elderly controls, EC) are able to compensate for the initial functional deficits by activating alternative cortical circuits in order to achieve correct execution of cognitive tasks [4, 5]. In particular, previous studies showed an age-related decrease in the responsiveness of parietal cortices during the successful performance of verbal, visual and spatial working memory tasks with a parallel recruitment of anterior frontal, cingulate and temporal cortices in normal brain aging [6, 7]. These changes might reflect brain efforts to counteract neurocognitive decline (compensation hypothesis). Using functional imaging, it has also been shown that high- but not low-performing elderly individuals may compensate for the age-related neural decline of parietal areas during working memory tasks, through the activation of distinct neurocognitive networks within prefrontal and limbic areas [6]. More recently, in their functional magnetic resonance imaging (fMRI) studies, Bodke et al. [8] and Yetkin et al. [9] also described functional compensation during face matching and working memory activation in MCI subjects. These observations suggest that the development of compensatory mechanisms takes place early in normal brain aging and may at least partly account for the metabolic differences observed between MCI and controls but also between MCI converters and nonconverters. With respect to pharmacological findings, two studies correlated levels of hippocampal choline acetyltransferase (ChAT) activity with the extent of AD lesions in control, MCI, and AD cases [10]. In contrast to that originally expected, MCI subjects presented with increased hippocampal ChAT activity and did not respond to the classic substitution therapy based on acetylcholinesterase inhibitors. This elevation was no longer present in mild AD cases, which were not different from controls. Severe AD cases showed markedly depleted hippocampal ChAT levels. Based on these observations, the authors postulated that cholinergic changes in the hippocampus of MCI subjects reflect a compensatory response to the progressive denervation of the hippocampus by lost entorhinal cortex input. It is thus likely that the earliest sign of subsequent cognitive decline is the functional breakdown of this compensation mainly in neocortical areas. Identifying functional changes in corticocortical circuits in MCI may thus allow to test in a near future the pertinence of predictive markers in cognitively intact individuals. Lastly, the use of simple and widely available imaging modalities is a key point in the identification of predictive markers of cognitive decline. Although clearly useful in research settings, PET and SPECT modalities show low temporal resolution (not necessarily compatible with the speed of functional compensation phenomena) and are thought to be invasive and not well accepted by elderly individuals. Despite its relevance for studying functional compensation phenomena, fMRI is rarely available in clinical settings.

The Role of Quantitative Electroencephalography

Electroencephalography (EEG) might be a powerful and simple tool for the identification of predictive markers of cognitive deterioration in MCI since it can investigate the rapid and multistage cognitive functions that are affected early in neurodegenerative processes with a high temporal resolution. Several previous EEG studies that focused on quantitative differences between healthy controls, MCI and AD cases led to conflicting results [11–16]. Early contributions reported altered theta-band relative power under rest conditions in AD compared to intellectually preserved individuals [17, 18], yet these observations have been later challenged [13, 16]. In follow-up studies of patients with mild AD or MCI, quantitative electroencephalographic data are predictive of further cognitive decline, yet the selected EEG parameters were highly variable. Among them, slow wave excess in the initial evaluation, decreased alpha and increased theta relative power and mean frequency in the left temporo-occipital region, and anteroposterior localization of alpha sources are the more consistent predictors of cognitive decline [14, 15]. However, cross-sectional comparisons revealed a substantial overlap in these parameters between MCI cases and EC raising doubts about their validity in routine clinical settings [12]. In particular, the limited sensitivity of these EEG analyses and absence of significant group differences in spectral EEG parameters [19] emphasize the necessity to use a cognitive activation design in such EEG investigations.

Electroencephalography Activation Studies

Since the evolution of AD is characterized by the progressive loss of functional connectivity within neocortical association areas, event-modulated EEG dynamic

Table 1. Distinction between PMCI and SMCI cases based on the three working memory load-dependent EEG hallmarks

	Sensitivity Pr(+| D)	Specificity Pr(-|~D)	Correctly classified
P200 latency (frontal site)	0.88	0.77	82.8%
N200 latency (frontal site)	0.75	0.69	72.4%
log% beta ERS (electrode P4)	0.56	0.69	62.1%
EEG signals combined	0.94	0.85	89.7%

analysis that makes it possible to investigate the functional activation of neocortical circuits, may represent a more sensitive method to identify early alterations of neuronal networks predictive of AD development among MCI cases. In fact, recent analyses identified changes of early endogenous event-related potentials and high beta frequency band reactivity in MCI or AD cases [3, 20]. In a very recent study attempting to investigate the usefulness of individual EEG activation parameters in the prediction of rapid cognitive decline in MCI, Missonnier et al. [21] focused on the analysis of three simple EEG parameters during the activation of working memory. They assessed P200 and N200 latencies as well as beta event-related synchronization (ERS) in 16 EC, 29 MCI cases and 10 patients with AD during the successful performance of a pure attentional detection task as compared to a highly working memory-demanding 2-back task. At 1-year follow-up, 16 MCI patients showed progressive cognitive decline (PMCI) and 13 remained stable (SMCI). Both P200 and N200 latencies in the 2-back task were longer in PMCI and AD cases compared to EC and SMCI cases. During the 1,000- to 1,700-ms interval after stimulus, beta ERS at parietal electrodes was of lower amplitude in PMCI and AD compared to EC and SMCI cases. Univariate models showed that P200, N200 and beta values were significantly related to the SMCI/PMCI distinction with areas under the receiver operating characteristic curve of 0.93, 0.78 and 0.72, respectively. The combination of all three EEG hallmarks was the stronger predictor of MCI deterioration with 90% of correctly classified MCI cases (table 1).

From a clinical viewpoint, the fact that PMCI cases behave as AD cases with respect to P200 and N200 latencies is a crucial step before using these individual EEG parameters in order to predict MCI conversion to AD. From a cognitive viewpoint and in agreement with recent functional imaging data [22, 23], this observation implies an impaired activation of the parietal generators involved in retrieval and storage phases of working memory activation in PMCI and AD. The sensitivity of high-frequency EEG oscillations to rapid cognitive decline is consistent with recent results from other

EEG and magnetoencephalography studies showing reduced beta reactivity in MCI and AD subjects as compared to elderly healthy controls in a working memory task [20]. The exact neurophysiological significance of this finding remains, however, a matter of debate. Recent lines of evidence indicated that synchronization of activities in high-frequency ranges may reflect the selective association of neurons distributed into functional groups [24]. In particular, beta ERS is known to increase during the retention period in a wide variety of active memory paradigms [25, 26]. The occurrence of beta ERS increase after the reaction time needed to compare incoming item and memory buffer suggests that it could be related to the active maintenance of new items for further task requirements [27]. Furthermore, the parietal location of beta energy observed in the present series is compatible with neuroimaging data showing that parietal areas are bilaterally engaged in storing verbal information in working memory [28]. Consistent with the previously described event-related potential findings, these observations provide additional evidence supporting the presence of early alterations of parietal generators involved in active maintenance of memory material for further task demands in PMCI and AD cases. The fact that PMCI and AD patients successfully completed the tasks despite these electrophysiological deficits indicates probable compensatory activation of additional cerebral areas. Accordingly, recent data suggest that high working memory performance can be maintained through the recruitment of alternative cortical networks even in the presence of early brain activation deficits in MCI [9].

New Perspectives

Despite the impressive progress with respect to the use of EEG as a tool for identification of early cortical dysfunctions in MCI groups, an individual prediction is still impossible. Inclusion of additional EEG markers may be a plausible strategy to ameliorate their predictive value in this context. However, one should keep in mind that the complexity of this approach should not obscure the main advantage of EEG that resides in its simple use in clinical settings. The choice of additional EEG marker is of particular relevance for activation studies. Although MCI has been initially conceptualized as a memory-related condition, the current theoretical models point to its heterogeneity related to the presence of several additional subtle cognitive deficits in this condition. Very recently, two studies attempted to identify early changes in the function of attentional circuits in MCI. The conceptual interest of their design resides in the focus on biological changes rather than overt cognitive deficits. In their fMRI study, Dannhauser et al. [29] reported early changes in the activation of dorsolateral prefrontal cortex in amnestic MCI cases during the successful performance of a divided attention paradigm (dual task). In line with the concept of functional compensation already described in MCI, these results suggested that the recruitment of alternative cortical circuits might allow for keeping high cognitive performance despite the presence of early deficits in brain activation. Within the same theoretical framework, Rosano et al. [4] analyzed by fMRI the activation of neocortical areas during the successful performance on the Preparing to Overcome Prepotency task, a classical executive control task. They reported that in contrast to EC that preferentially activated dorsolateral prefrontal and anterior cingulate cortex, MCI cases activated the posterior parietal cortex in the context of a compensatory reallocation of cognitive resources. The authors suggested that this preferential activation of the posterior parietal cortex represents the first line of defense in order to keep stable performances in MCI. Unfortunately, the cross-sectional design of the study did not allow us to draw conclusions about the significance of posterior parietal cortex activation as a possible predictive marker of further cognitive decline. Future EEG activation studies exploring the brain reactivity during the performance of attentional/executive function tests may lead to the identification of new predictive markers corresponding to MCI subgroups.

The second theoretical issue concerns the prediction of cognitive decline in normal elderly individuals. Following the well-established idea that individuals with MCI compensate via the activation of alternative cortical circuits the presence of an already substantial biological compromise, one can reasonably doubt about the usefulness of future curative strategies in this population. From this point of view, the identification of EEG markers able to predict cognitive deterioration in the entorhinal cortex is a key step towards the establishment of effective interventions or preventive strategies at the earliest possible time. To date, there is only one prospective study of normal elders with subjective complaints indicating that quantitative EEG data such as increase in theta power, slowing of mean frequency and decreased coherence between the right central and posterior regions at baseline may accurately predict future cognitive decline during 7- to 9-year follow-up [30]. Replication of these findings and additional longitudinal data regarding EEG activation parameters may provide future tools for an appropriate screening of normal elderly individuals prone to develop cognitive decline. However, a wide application of an EEG-based screening for trait markers of future deterioration in old age presents several problems. First, the number of decliners may be to low to obtain significant results especially in short follow-up periods. Second, although conceptually more appropriate, long follow-up in limited series might lead to positive data that reflect selection biases without real biological significance (i.e. it is difficult to establish a clear relationship between EEG patterns at baseline and MCI-related structural and functional changes after one decade). To address this problem, two strategies may be considered. The first implicates the performance of long-term follow-up in large community-based series that guarantee a sufficient number of decliners and absence (or at least relative rarity) of selection biases. Alternatively, one could isolate subsamples of normal elderly people carrying risk factors for dementia based on their genetic and biochemical profile. After this initial screening, EEG parameters at baseline may have greater chance to be predictive of cognitive decline even during a short-term follow-up. In this respect, a recent multicentric EEG study revealed an association between the presence of the ε4 allele of apolipoprotein E and amplitude of alpha 1 and 2 sources in limbic areas, further stressing the interest of genotype-EEG phenotype studies in the early prediction of AD [31]. Keeping in mind that EEG analysis represents an objective, cost-effective, culture-fair, noninvasive evaluation method, the combination of these two strategies may provide us in a near future with new sensitive tools for the identification of individuals at high risk for dementia among cognitively intact elders. Should this first step be successful, one could oversee later on an EEG-based individual prediction of dementia risk.

References

1 DeCarli C: Mild cognitive impairment: prevalence, prognosis, aetiology, and treatment. Lancet Neurol 2003;2:15–21.

2 Petersen RC, Doody R, Kurz A, Mohs RC, Morris JC, Rabins PV, Ritchie K, Rossor M, Thal L, Winblad B: Current concepts in mild cognitive impairment. Arch Neurol 2001;58:1985–1992.

3 Missonnier P, Gold G, Fazio-Costa L, Michel JP, Mulligan R, Michon A, Ibáñez V, Giannakopoulos P: Early event-related potential changes during working memory activation predict rapid decline in mild cognitive impairment. J Gerontol A Biol Sci Med Sci 2005;60:660–666.

4 Rosano C, Aizenstein HJ, Cochran JL, Saxton JA, De Kosky ST, Newman AB, Kuller LH, Lopez OL, Carter CS: Event-related functional magnetic resonance imaging investigation of executive control in very old individuals with mild cognitive impairment. Biol Psychiatry 2005;57:761–767.

5 Thulborn KR, Martin C, Voyvodic JT: Functional MR imaging using a visually guided saccade paradigm for comparing activation patterns in patients with probable Alzheimer's disease and in cognitively able elderly volunteers. Am J Neuroradiol 2000;21: 524–531.

6 Cabeza R, Dolcos F, Graham R, Nyberg L: Similarities and differences in the neural correlates of episodic memory retrieval and working memory. Neuroimage 2002;16:317–330.

7 McEvoy LK, Pellouchoud E, Smith ME, Gevins A: Neurophysiological signals of working memory in normal aging. Cogn Brain Res 2001;11:363–376.

8 Bokde AL, Lopez-Bayo P, Meindl T, Pechler S, Born C, Faltraco F, Teipel SJ, Moller HJ, Hampel H: Functional connectivity of the fusiform gyrus during a face-matching task in subjects with mild cognitive impairment. Brain 2006;129:1113–1124.

9 Yetkin FZ, Rosenberg RN, Weiner MF, Purdy PD, Cullum CM: fMRI of working memory in patients with mild cognitive impairment and probable Alzheimer's disease. Eur Radiol 2006;16:193–206.

10 Ikonomovic MD, Mufson EJ, Wuu J, Cochran EJ, Bennett DA, DeKosky ST: Cholinergic plasticity in hippocampus of individuals with mild cognitive impairment: correlation with Alzheimer's neuropathology. J Alzheimers Dis 2003;5:39–48.

11 Cichocki A, Shishkin SL, Musha T, Leonowicz Z, Asada T, Kurachi T: EEG filtering based on blind source separation (BSS) for early detection of Alzheimer's disease. Clin Neurophysiol 2005;116: 729–737.

12 Frodl T, Hampel H, Juckel G, Burger K, Padberg F, Engel RR, Moller HJ, Hegerl U: Value of event-related P300 subcomponents in the clinical diagnosis of mild cognitive impairment and Alzheimer's disease. Psychophysiology 2002;39:175–181.

13 Grunwald M, Busse F, Hensel A, Riedel-Heller S, Kruggel F, Arendt T, Wolf H, Gertz HJ: Theta-power differences in patients with mild cognitive impairment under rest condition and during haptic tasks. Alzheimer Dis Assoc Disord 2002;16:40–48.

14 Huang C, Wahlund L, Dierks T, Julin P, Winblad B, Jelic V: Discrimination of Alzheimer's disease and mild cognitive impairment by equivalent EEG sources: a cross-sectional and longitudinal study. Clin Neurophysiol 2000;111:1961–1967.

15 Jelic V, Johansson SE, Almkvist O, Shigeta M, Julin P, Nordberg A, Winblad B, Wahlund LO: Quantitative electroencephalography in mild cognitive impairment: longitudinal changes and possible prediction of Alzheimer's disease. Neurobiol Aging 2000;21:533–540.

16 Stam CJ, van der Made Y, Pijnenburg YA, Scheltens P: EEG synchronization in mild cognitive impairment and Alzheimer's disease. Acta Neurol Scand 2003;108:90–96.
17 Jelic V, Dierks T, Amberla K, Almkvist O, Winblad B, Nordberg A: Longitudinal changes in quantitative EEG during long-term tacrine treatment of patients with Alzheimer's disease. Neurosci Lett 1998; 254:85–88.
18 Signorino M, Pucci E, Belardinelli N, Nolfe G, Angeleri F: EEG spectral analysis in vascular and Alzheimer dementia. Electroencephalogr Clin Neurophysiol 1995;94:313–325.
19 Gunther W, Giunta R, Klages U, Haag C, Steinberg R, Satzger W, Jonitz L, Engel R: Findings of electroencephalographic brain mapping in mild to moderate dementia of the Alzheimer type during resting, motor, and music-perception conditions. Psychiatry Res 1993;50:163–176.
20 Karrasch M, Laine M, Rinne JO, Rapinoja P, Sinerva E, Krause CM: Brain oscillatory responses to an auditory-verbal working memory task in mild cognitive impairment and Alzheimer's disease. Int J Psychophysiol 2006;59:168–178.
21 Missonnier P, Deiber MP, Gold G, Herrmann FR, Millet P, Michon A, Fazio-Costa L, Ibanez V, Giannakopoulos P: Working memory load-related electroencephalographic parameters can differentiate progressive from stable mild cognitive impairment. Neuroscience 2007;150:346–356.
22 Drzezga A, Lautenschlager N, Siebner H, Riemenschneider M, Willoch F, Minoshima S, Schwaiger M, Kurz A: Cerebral metabolic changes accompanying conversion of mild cognitive impairment into Alzheimer's disease: a PET follow-up study. Eur J Nucl Med Mol Imaging 2003;30:1104–1113.
23 Huang C, Wahlund LO, Almkvist O, Elehu D, Svensson L, Jonsson T, Winblad B, Julin P: Voxel- and VOI-based analysis of SPECT CBF in relation to clinical and psychological heterogeneity of mild cognitive impairment. Neuroimage 2003;19:1137–1144.
24 Varela F, Lachaux JP, Rodriguez E, Martinerie J: The brainweb: phase synchronization and large-scale integration. Nat Rev Neurosci 2001;2:229–239.
25 Onton J, Delorme A, Makeig S: Frontal midline EEG dynamics during working memory. Neuroimage 2005;27:341–356.
26 Ravizza SM, Behrmann M, Fiez JA: Right parietal contributions to verbal working memory: spatial or executive? Neuropsychologia 2005;43:2057–2067.
27 Deiber MP, Missonnier P, Bertrand O, Gold G, Fazio-Costa L, Ibáñez V, Giannakopoulos P: Distinction between perceptual and attentional processing in working memory tasks: a study of phase-locked and induced oscillatory brain dynamics. J Cogn Neurosci 2007;19:158–172.
28 Cohen JD, Perlstein WM, Braver TS, Nystrom LE, Noll DC, Jonides J, Smith EE: Temporal dynamics of brain activation during a working memory task. Nature 1997;386:604–608.
29 Dannhauser TM, Walker Z, Stevens T, Lee L, Seal M, Shergill SS: The functional anatomy of divided attention in amnestic mild cognitive impairment. Brain 2005;128:1418–1427.
30 Prichep LS, John ER, Ferris SH, Rausch L, Fang Z, Cancro R, Torossian C, Reisberg B: Prediction of longitudinal cognitive decline in normal elderly with subjective complaints using electrophysiological imaging. Neurobiol Aging 2006;27:471–481.
31 Babiloni C, Benussi L, Binetti G, Cassetta E, Dal Forno G, Del Percio C, Ferreri F, Ferri R, Frisoni G, Ghidoni R, Miniussi C, Rodriguez G, Romani GL, Squitti R, Ventriglia MC, Rossini PM: Apolipoprotein E and alpha brain rhythms in mild cognitive impairment: a multicentric electroencephalogram study. Ann Neurol 2006;59:323–334.

Prof. Panteleimon Giannakopoulos
Division of Geriatric Psychiatry, Department of Psychiatry
University of Geneva School of Medicine
2, chemin du Petit-Bel-Air
CH–1225 Chêne-Bourg, Geneva (Switzerland)
Tel. +41 22 305 5001, Fax +41 22 305 5044
E-Mail Panteleimon.Giannakopoulos@medecine.unige.ch

Giannakopoulos P, Hof PR (eds): Dementia in Clinical Practice.
Front Neurol Neurosci. Basel, Karger, 2009, vol 24, pp 47–53

The Future: New Methods of Imaging Exploration in Alzheimer's Disease

Agneta Nordberg

Department of Neurobiology, Care Sciences and Society, Karolinska Institutet, and Division of Alzheimer Neurobiology, Department of Geriatric Medicine, Karolinska University Hospital Huddinge, Stockholm, Sweden

Abstract

Alzheimer's disease (AD) is a complex disease characterized by a whole cascade of pathological events. During the last 100 years, the role of amyloid in the development of AD has been the focus of major research. Today there is hope that amyloid imaging may help in the early detection of the disease and be used for evaluating new drug therapies including neuroprotective and preventive therapies in AD. The rapid development of the molecular imaging techniques now allows in vivo imaging not only of brain functional activity such as cerebral blood flow, cerebral glucose metabolism and neurotransmitter activity, and receptor density, but also pathological processes such as amyloid plaques and microglial activation in AD. Several positron emission tomography amyloid imaging ligands have recently been developed and tested in AD patients. High amyloid content can be detected in vivo by positron emission tomography in prodromal AD preceding the impairment of functional activity like cerebral glucose metabolism, and reduction in cholinergic activity, which are likely to follow the course of cognitive impairment.

Since their description in Alois Alzheimer's classical paper 'Über eine eigenartige Erkrankung der Hirnrinde' in 1907, the presence of senile plaques and neurofibrillary tangles has been considered as the classical neuropathological hallmark of Alzheimer's disease (AD). β-Amyloid (Aβ) appears to deposit in the brain earlier in the course of the disease than the appearance of neurofibrillary tangles, which seem to be more closely related to impairment in neurotransmission. Whether amyloid is the primary cause of AD has however not yet been proven. It is nonetheless quite apparent that a whole cascade of events is triggered in the brain following the appearance of abnormal levels of amyloid in brain [1, 2]. A complicating factor for the understanding of the Aβ pathology is the existence of multiple forms of Aβ from monomers and oligomers to fibrils forming the insoluble amyloid plaques. The positive news is that we can measure amyloid plaques in vivo by imaging the brain of AD patients [3]. The oligomers in the brain might be more toxic than the amyloid plaques, triggering synaptic failure and inducing inflammatory processes [4], and today it is still impossible to measure oligomers in the brain of living patients perhaps due to quite low concentrations and higher solubility.

There has been a rapid development in both structural and functional imaging, allowing in vivo measurement of brain disturbances in AD patients. Structural imaging technologies such as computed tomography and magnetic resonance imaging provide important information about brain structures for the diagnosis of dementia, while an insight into brain functional activity has been provided by single photon emission tomography and especially positron emission tomography (PET). Changes in cerebral blood flow and cerebral glucose metabolism have been demonstrated in AD and patients with mild cognitive impairment (MCI) [5, 6]. New molecular imaging tracers for imaging of various pathological processes will provide a deeper insight into various molecular processes that are ongoing in AD. By developing surrogate markers in AD, they can be used as early diagnostic tools as well as in the evaluation of new therapeutic treatments. Table 1 illustrates tracers used for molecular imaging studies visualizing different pathological processes and neurotransmitter functions in AD.

Neurochemical Imaging of Cholinergic Neurotransmission in Alzheimer's Disease

AD is characterized by changes in neurotransmitter functions that seem to correlate with impairment in the cognitive function typical for the disease. The prominent role of the cholinergic system in cognitive functions and AD has contributed to the development of PET tracers for measurement of the enzyme acetylcholinesterase (AChE) as well as ligands for muscarinic and nicotinic receptors [7, 8].

AChE activity in AD brains has been mapped by PET and the radiolabeled acetylcholine analogues, N-[^{11}C]-methyl-piperidine-4-yl-propionate (^{11}C-PMP) and N-[^{11}C]-methyl-piperidine-4-yl-acetate (^{11}C-MP4A) [9]. A lower AChE activity has been measured in cortical brain regions of MCI patients who later converted to AD [10]. A higher AChE activity has been measured using ^{11}C-MP4A and PET in ApoE $\varepsilon 4$ carriers compared to ApoE $\varepsilon 4$ noncarriers [11]. A significant correlation between attention tests such as digit span and cortical AChE activity, measured by ^{11}C-PMP, has been described in AD patients [12]. Furthermore, a significant positive correlation was observed between the degree of AChE inhibition and improvement in digit span test in mild AD patients treated with galantamine for 12 months [13].

There is a loss of nicotinic receptors in the brain of AD patients. PET studies using ^{11}C-nicotine have demonstrated that the loss in ^{11}C-nicotine binding significantly correlates with cognition, as measured by Mini-Mental State Examination [14]. Recently, Kadir et al. [15] showed a significant correlation between ^{11}C-nicotine binding in the frontal and parietal cortices and the results of attention test such as digit symbol and trail making test. A positive correlation was also found between increase in ^{11}C-nicotine binding and improvement in digit span test following long-term treatment

Table 1. Tracers used for molecular imaging

Neurotransmission	Imaging tracers
Cholinergic system	
Nicotinic receptors	^{11}C-nicotine, ^{18}F-A855380
Muscarinic receptors	^{11}C-NMPB
AChE	^{11}C-PMP, ^{11}C-MP4A
Serotonergic system	
Serotonin receptors	
$5HT_{1A}$	^{11}C-WAY, ^{11}C-MPFF
$5HT_{2A}$	^{11}C-altanserin
Dopaminergic system	
Dopamine D2 receptors	^{11}C-raclopride
DOPA transporter	^{11}C-FP-CIT
DOPA decarboxylation	^{18}F-fluorodopa
GABA system	
GABA receptors	^{11}C-flumazenil
Amyloid plaques	^{18}F-FDNNP
	^{11}C-PIB
	^{11}C-SB13
	^{18}F-BF-227
	^{18}F-BAY94-9172
	^{18}F-AV-144
Microglial activation	^{11}C-PK-11195
Astrocytes	^{11}C-Deprenyl

with rivastigmine and galantamine [15, 16]. Molecular imaging of AChE activity and ^{11}C-nicotine binding have thus revealed changes during cholinesterase inhibitor treatment corresponding to the measured outcome in cognitive performance as attention tests in AD patients. It will probably be necessary in the future of drug development to focus more on molecular imaging studies than solely on large clinical trials with cognitive tests as outcome measures for new drug identification in AD.

Amyloid Imaging in Alzheimer's Disease

The development of plaque-binding compounds started 15 years ago by testing whether monoclonal antibodies against Aβ as well as peptide fragments could be

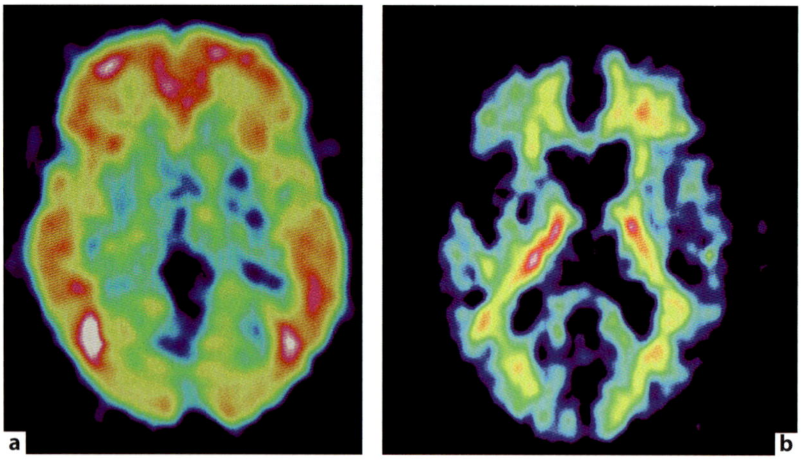

Fig. 1. **a** Amyloid load in large cortical brain regions of an AD patient as measured with ^{11}C-PIB and PET. **b** Similar studies performed in an age-matched healthy control show low PIB retention in brain. The color scales correspond to red = high, yellow = moderate, green = low, blue = very low. Photos from Uppsala PET Centre/Imanet and Karolinska University Hospital Huddinge.

used for imaging amyloid in brain [3]. These attempts failed due to the poor penetrations of the tracer ligands into the brain. More promising were the strategies of using small radiolabeled analogues of Congo red, chrysamine-G, and thioflavin applicable to single photon emission tomography and PET [3]. Table 1 illustrates the different ^{11}C and ^{18}F compounds that have been used so far for amyloid imaging in AD. Figure 1 shows high amyloid load in AD brain compared to control as measured by ^{11}C-PIB and PET.

^{18}F-FDDNP was the first amyloid ligand studied in AD patients in 2002 [17] followed by ^{11}C-PIB in 2004 [18]. Opposite to ^{11}C-PIB, ^{18}F-FDDNP was reported to bind also to neurofibrillary tangles in the brain [19]. The first ^{11}C-PIB studies were performed in a group of Swedish mild AD patients showing significantly higher PIB retention in the frontal, temporal, parietal, and occipital cortices and the striatum (1.9–1.5 times differences) compared to healthy controls [18]. The retention of ^{11}C-PIB was low and comparable in the pons and cerebellum of AD patients and healthy controls [18]. These observations with ^{11}C-PIB [18] have later been confirmed by several research groups [for review, see 20]. It is estimated that more than 2,000 subjects now have been scanned with the PIB PET amyloid imaging ligand worldwide [Klunk, pers. commun.]. Studies have now also been performed with other amyloid ligands such as ^{11}C-SB-13 [21], ^{18}F-BF-227 [22], and ^{18}F-BAY94-9172 [23]. ^{18}F-BF-227 appears to be somewhat more sensitive in the later stage of disease [22]. Rowe et al. [23] concluded when comparing ^{18}F-BAY94-9172 with ^{11}C-PIB that ^{18}F-BAY94-9172 showed 57% higher binding in the cortex of AD patients compared to healthy controls, whereas ^{11}C-PIB showed 70% higher binding in AD cortex compared to healthy controls [23]. The labeling with ^{18}F compared to ^{11}C may have some advantage allowing a broader clinical application of the amyloid tracers.

A 2-year follow-up study with PIB showed no significant change in PIB retention compared to baseline despite that all AD patients showed a decline in cerebral glucose metabolism and some of the patients a measurable reduction in cognitive function of more than 3 points in Mini-Mental State Examination at follow-up period [24]. The unchanged PIB retention on 2-year follow-up scans suggests a different time course for amyloid load in comparison to changes in functional activity in the brain.

MCI is considered as a transitional state between normal aging and AD. High ^{11}C-PIB retention has been demonstrated in MCI patients compared to healthy controls and some MCI patients show as high PIB retention as AD patients [25]. A significant negative correlation has been observed between cortical ^{11}C-PIB retention and $A\beta_{1-42}$ levels in cerebrospinal fluid (CSF), and a positive correlation between ^{11}C-PIB retention and CSF tau in MCI patients [25]. The findings suggest that amyloid imaging with ^{11}C-PIB in addition to CSF biomarkers may allow early detection of prodromal AD.

Brain Amyloid Imaging and Cognition

It is well established from several studies in autopsy brain tissue from AD patients that the amount of amyloid plaque pathology appears to correlate less with cognitive function than neurofibrillary tangles and neurotransmitter activity. So far, the in vivo amyloid imaging studies have shown a negative correlation between episodic memory test score and cortical ^{11}C-PIB retention in MCI and AD patients [24–26]. Pike et al. [26] found a strong correlation between episodic memory and ^{11}C-PIB binding for MCI patients, while the same correlation was weak for AD patients [26], which again emphasizes the differences in time-course that might exist between amyloid load in the brain and impairment of functional brain activity in AD.

The presence of amyloid plaques has been reported at autopsy in the cerebral cortex of cognitive normal older subjects and positive 'amyloid signal' has also been observed with ^{11}C-PIB [20, 27, 28], as well as with ^{18}F-BAY94-9172 [23]. It is estimated that the amyloid might be present in 30% of normal elderly subjects [28]. Whether these normal elderly subjects will develop in AD later on has yet to be systematically investigated, and it is necessary to find other factors with a possible preventive effect.

Amyloid Imaging and Anti-Amyloid Therapy

At present, there is a great focus on the development of different drugs interacting with the amyloid processes in AD including APP (amyloid precursor protein) processing, Aβ aggregation and elimination. Different targets include inhibition of β- and γ-secretases or modulation of γ-secretase, inhibition of Aβ fibrillation, reducing Aβ accumulation, and increasing removal of Aβ plaques. Different active and passive immunization therapies are ongoing worldwide in AD patients. In vivo amyloid imaging prior and following immunization therapy would therefore preferably be performed in treated AD patients in order to verify the reduction in amyloid in patients after immunization.

Phenserine, an inhibitor of the formation of βAPP in addition to its cholinesterase inhibitor effect is probably the first drug where the effect on ^{11}C-PIB retentions has been followed during 6 months' treatment of mild AD patients [29]. The obtained data suggest that phenserine treatment can influence both the amyloid content in the brain as well as in CSF together with an improvement in cognition [29]. Further PET amyloid studies will provide a deeper understanding of the underlying mechanisms for antiamyloid therapy.

Imaging of Microglial Activation

Studies with PET ligands such as ^{11}C-PK-11195 as markers for microglial activation in the brain have shown higher binding in AD patients compared to age-matched healthy controls as a sign for microglia activation in different parts of the AD brain [30]. Further studies are needed to investigate the relationship between microglial activation and amyloid load decrease in cerebral glucose metabolism and cognition. It will also be important to study these nonneuronal cell processes following amyloid immunization therapies.

Acknowledgement

The financial support of the Swedish Research Council (project No. 05817), Stohnes Foundation, Foundation of Old Servants, KI Foundations, The Alzheimer Foundation in Sweden, Brain Foundation, Swedish Brain Power, and the EC-FP6 project DiMI, LSHB-CT-2005-512146, QLK6-CT-2000-00502 is gratefully acknowledged.

References

1 Hardy JA, Selkoe DJ: The amyloid hypothesis of Alzheimer's disease: progress and problems on the road to therapeutics. Science 2002;297:353–356.

2 Mattson MP: Pathways towards and away from Alzheimer's disease. Nature 2004;430:631–639.

3 Nordberg A: PET imaging of amyloid in Alzheimer's disease. Lancet Neurol 2004;3:519–527.

4 Selkoe DJ: Alzheimer's disease is a synaptic failure. Science 2002;298:789–791.

5 Herholz K, Carter SF, Jones M: Positron emission tomography imaging in dementia. Br J Radiology 2007;80:S160–S167.

6 Small G, Brooksheimer SY, Thompson PM, Cole GM, Huang SC, Kepe V, Barrio JR: Current and future uses of neuroimaging for cognitively impaired patients. Lancet Neurol 2008;7:161–172.

7 Nordberg A: Visualization of nicotinic and muscarinic receptors in brain by positron emission tomography; in Giacobini E, Pepeu G (eds): The Cholinergic System in Health and Disease. London, Informa Healthcare, 2006, pp 181–190.
8 Långström B, Andrén PE, Lindhe O, Svedberg M, Hall H: In vitro imaging techniques in neurodegenerative diseases. Mol Imaging Biol 2007;9:161–175.
9 Kuhl DE, Koeppe RA, Minoshima S, et al: In vivo mapping of cerebral acetylcholinesterase activity in aging and Alzheimer's disease. Neurology 1999; 52:691–699.
10 Herholz K, Weisenbach S, Kalbe E, et al: Cerebral acetylcholine esterase activity in mild cognitive impairment. Neuroreport 2005;16:1431–1434.
11 Eggers C, Herlholz K, Kalbe E, Heiss WD: Cortical acetylcholine esterase activity and ApoE4-genotype in Alzheimer's disease. Neurosci Lett 2006;408: 46–50.
12 Bohnen NI, Kaufer DI, Hendrickson R, et al: Cognitive correlates of alterations in acetylcholinesterase in Alzheimer's disease. Neurosci Lett 2005; 380:127–132.
13 Kadir A, Darreh-Shori T, Almkvist O, et al: PET imaging of the in vivo brain acetylcholinesterase activity and nicotine binding in galantamine-treated patients with AD. Neurobiol Aging 2008;29: 1204–1217.
14 Nordberg A, Lundqvist H, Hartvig P, et al: Kinetic analysis of regional (S)(-)^{11}C-nicotine binding in normal and Alzheimer brains. In vivo assessments using positron emission tomography. Alzh Dis Assoc Disord 1995;9:21–27.
15 Kadir A, Almkvist O, Wall A, Långström B, Nordberg A: PET imaging of cortical ^{11}C-nicotine binding correlates with the cognitive function of attention in Alzheimer's diseases. Psychopharmacology 2006;188:509–520.
16 Kadir A, Darreh-Shori T, Almkvist O, Wall A, Långström B, Nordberg A: Changes in brain (^{11}C)-nicotine binding sites in patients with mild Alzheimer's disease following rivastigmine treatment as assessed by PET. Psychopharmacology 2007;191:1005–1014.
17 Shoghi-Jadid K, Small D, Agdeppa ED, et al: Localization of neurofibrillary tangles and beta-amyloid plaques in the brain of living patients with Alzheimer disease. Am J Geriat Psychiatry 2002;10: 24–35.
18 Klunk WE, Engler H, Nordberg A, et al: Imaging brain amyloid in Alzheimer's disease with Pittsburgh compound B. Ann Neurol 2004;55:306–319.
19 Ye L, Morgenstern JL, Gee AD: Delineation of PET imaging agent binding sites on beta-amyloid peptide fibrils. J Biol Chem 2005;280:23599–23604.
20 Nordberg A: Amyloid imaging in Alzheimer's disease. Neuropsychologia 2008;46:1636–1641.
21 Verhoeff NP, Wilson AA, Takeshita S, et al: In vivo imaging of Alzheimer disease beta-amyloid with [^{11}C]SB-13 PET. J Am Geriat Psychiatry 2004;12: 584–595.
22 Kudo Y, Okamura N, Furumoto S, et al: 2-(2-[2-Dimethylaminothiazol-5-yl] ethenyl)-6-(2-[fluoro] ethoxy)benzoxazole: a novel PET agent for in vivo detection of dense amyloid plaques in Alzheimer's disease patients. J Nucl Med 2007;48: 553–561.
23 Rowe CC, Ackerman U, Browne W, et al: Imaging of amyloid β in Alzheimer's disease with 18F-BAY94-9172, a novel PET tracer: proof of mechanism. Lancet Neurol 2008;7:129–135.
24 Engler H, Forsberg A, Almkvist O, et al: Two year follow-up of amyloid deposition in patients with Alzheimer's disease. Brain 2006;12:2856–2866.
25 Forsberg A, Engler H, Almkvist O, et al: PET imaging of amyloid deposition in patients with mild cognitive impairment. Neurobiol Aging 2008;29: 1456–1465.
26 Pike KE, Savage G, Villemagne VL, et al: β-Amyloid imaging and memory in non-demented individuals: evidence for preclinical Alzheimer's disease. Brain 2007;130:2037–2844.
27 Mintun MA, LaRosso GN, Dence CS, et al: [^{11}C] PIB in a nondement population. Potential antecendent marker of Alzheimer's disease. Neurology 2006;67:446–452.
28 Villemagne VL, Pike KE, Darby D, et al: Aβ deposition in older non-demented individuals with cognitive decline are indicative of preclinical Alzheimer's disease. Neuropsychologia 2008;46:1688–1697.
29 Kadir A, Andreasen N, Almkvist O, et al: Effect of phenserine treatment on brain functional activity and amyloid in AD. Ann Neurol 2008;63:621–631.
30 Cagnin A Brooks DJ, Kennedy AM, et al: In vivo measurement of activated microglia in dementia. Lancet 2001;358:461–467.

Prof. Agneta Nordberg, MD, PhD
Karolinska Institutet, Department of Neurobiology
Care Sciences and Society, Division of Alzheimer Neurobiology
Karolinska University Hospital Huddinge, Novum 5th floor, SE–141 86 Stockholm (Sweden)
Tel. +46 8 5858 5467, Fax 46 8 5858 5470, E-Mail Agneta.K.Nordberg@ki.se

Giannakopoulos P, Hof PR (eds): Dementia in Clinical Practice.
Front Neurol Neurosci. Basel, Karger, 2009, vol 24, pp 54–65

Pharmacological Interventions in Primary Care: Hopes and Illusions

Frédéric Assal · Marian van der Meulen

Department of Clinical Neurosciences, Faculty of Medicine and Neurology,
University Hospitals of Geneva, Geneva, Switzerland

Abstract

Alzheimer's disease is a neurodegenerative disease characterized by senile plaques, neurofibrillary tangles, synaptic loss, neuronal death and cholinergic deficits, causing cognitive, behavioral and psychological deficits, as well as a functional impairment that results in serious caregiver distress and a great economic burden worldwide. High hopes rose with the development of symptomatic treatments, resulting from randomized controlled trials using cholinergic enhancers or cholinesterase inhibitors, such as donepezil, galantamine and rivastigmine. When memantine, an NMDA antagonist, was approved and the first phase III antiamyloid immunization was launched, many clinicians eagerly anticipated the first disease-modifying drugs in their daily practice. For the treatment of behavioral and psychological symptoms of dementia (BPSD), atypical antipsychotics and new-generation antidepressants also seemed to offer great promises, mainly because of their good tolerance and side effect profiles. Hopes, however, were followed by desillusions: subsequent studies demonstrated that cholinesterase inhibitors and memantine had only modest and short-lived effects on cognition and BPSD, and the effect of antipsychotics on BPSD appeared questionable. Disease-modifying drugs such as antiamyloid immunization or amyloid clearance medication had to be abandoned for safety reasons or absence of efficacy. Although the early treatment of vascular risk factors is increasingly recognized in Alzheimer's disease prevention because of their implication in the amyloid cascade, randomized controlled trials have yielded largely negative results. Therefore, pharmacological as well as fundamental research that better underpins the complex pathophysiology of this devastating disease constitutes one of the biggest challenges of the 21st century.

Alzheimer's disease (AD) is clinically defined as an impairment in memory, as well as in a second cognitive domain, resulting in significant functional decline as assessed with measures of instrumental and basic activities of daily living (ADL) [1]. Various neuropsychological instruments ranging from brief bedside mental state screening scales to extensive neuropsychological batteries have been developed to diagnose, follow-up and/or compare patients under medication. In trials of AD treatments, most federal regulations require two outcome criteria in order to demonstrate the clinical relevance of the drug-placebo difference, namely improvement of the core cognitive deficit (usually assessed with the ADAS-cog) and improvement of a global or functional measure. In the past decade, neuropsychiatric or behavioral and psychological symptoms in dementia (BPSD) have been increasingly recognized as part of the disease [for review, see 2]. BPSD such as depression, anxiety, apathy, delusions, agitation and aggression are common in AD, frequently occur in combination, are demanding for caregivers and lead to nursing home placement. Often, however, these symptoms do not meet the criteria for diagnosis of the same phenomenological symptoms consistent with psychiatric diseases. Therefore, important psychotropic drugs approved for psychiatric diseases have not been tested and are usually not approved for BPSD in AD by most countries.

Using the results from systematic meta-analyses, reviews, main randomized controlled trials (RCTs) and expert opinions, we review treatments that were very promising when they were introduced, but that have been challenged more recently, sometimes even showing null effects in RCTs. The current main treatments are discussed from the primary care physicians' (PCPs) perspective, since physicians represent key figures in AD care in most countries. This review will present our hopes and illusions and give some practical recommendations on treatments that may alleviate cognitive and noncognitive symptoms of this devastating disease.

See Practical Recommendations, and table 1 for main drug treatment dosage.

Practical Recommendations

When and how to refer to a specialist or a memory clinic is a crucial question for PCPs and depends on many different factors, such as the expertise of the PCP, availability of specialists and, in several countries, federal regulations (i.e. some specifically require certain treatments to be prescribed by specialists only). Referring all patients with dementia would not be cost effective and specialists might get overbooked rapidly. Generally, the main reasons for referral are early dementia in professionally active persons (when it is ruled out that the symptoms are caused by normal aging, depression or anxiety), young-onset dementia, the presence of strong family history, and non-AD dementias. The classical red flags for non-AD dementia are early behavioral symptoms, such as disinhibition, profound apathy, hallucinations, neurological signs such as parkinsonism, cerebellar indications, gait problems and focal deficits or neuroimaging findings, such as abnormal T2 hyperintensities, focal atrophy, or normal pressure hydrocephalus suspicion. Other reasons for referral may be second opinion, little or no response to cholinesterase inhibitors (ChEIns) or memantine, unusual side effects, or difficult neuropsychiatric symptoms.

Cholinesterase Inhibitors

Apart from neurofibrillary tangles, senile plaque formation, and neuronal and synaptic loss, a profound reduction in cholinergic neurotransmission, secondary to

Table 1. Current medications used in AD

		Indication	Starting dose	Maintenance dose (daily)	Main side-effects (SE)	Remarks	Future directions
ChEIns	Donepezil	Mild to moderate stage	5 mg qs	10 mg qs (increased after 4 weeks)	Gastrointestinal (GI) Bradycardia, heart block	Efficacy appears similar and choice mainly depends on PCP experience and patient tolerance MCI: no consensus but a trial of donepezil could be proposed	Head-to-head comparisons Better define responders vs. nonresponders
	Galantamine		8 mg qs (with meals)	16 (24) mg qs after 4 (8) weeks	Same as above		
	Rivastigmine		1.5 mg bid (with meals) Patch 5–10 (20 in the US)	Increase in 2nd week 3 mg daily increment Low dosage for 4 weeks then increase	Same as above, GI more marked GI less prominent than with capsule		
Anti-NMDA blockers	Memantine	Moderate to severe stage	10–20	4-week titration 10 mg bid	Dizziness, confusion, drowsiness, hallucinations	Easier titration (two steps) and once-daily possible Rapid switch from ChEIns possible Might be beneficial in agitation	Comparisons with ChEIns
Antipsychotics	*Conventional*: Haloperidol (H), Thioridazine, Chlorpromazine	Extreme agitation Acute psychosis	0.5 mg im	0.5–1 mg (try to avoid)	High sedation Extrapyramidal symptoms QT prolongation	If BPSD (psychosis, agitation) are modest, try first with ChEIns or memantine H im if extreme agitation and for very short periods Q or C if extrapyramidal signs are present before treatment C: monitor leukocytes	More comparisons with atypical antipsychotics More head-to-head comparisons New agents with better SE profile
	Olanzapine (O)	Delusions Agitation	2.5 mg	2.5–5 mg	Same as above Fewer extrapyramidal symptoms especially for Q and C C: Agranulocytosis		
	Risperidone (R)		0.5 mg	0.5–1 mg			
	Quietapine (Q)		12.5–25 mg qs	25–150 mg			
	Clozapine (C)		12.5 mg qs	25–100 mg			

Table 1. Continued

		Indication	Starting dose	Maintenance dose (daily)	Main side-effects (SE)	Remarks	Future directions
Antidepressants	Citalopram	Depression Agitation	10–20 mg	20–40 mg qs	Agitation, tremor, anorexia, nausea, drowsiness More rarely serotoninergic syndrome		
	Sertraline	Particularly with insomnia	50 mg	50 (100) mg bid			
	Trazodone		25–50 mg	50–200 mg in one of 2 doses			
Others	Carbamazepine Valproate acid	No evidence, should be abandoned, cave confusion and hyponatremia with carbamazepine, confusion, ataxia, tremor with valproate					
	Gabapentin	Agitation, anxiety (?)	100 mg	300–2,400 mg	Sedation	No dependence	Need for RCT
	Benzodiazepine i.e. Lorazepam	Acute stressful condition	1–2.5 mg	Try to avoid	Sedation, memory loss, falls, paradoxical reaction, dependence		

(1) Neurologists, geriatricians, psychiatrists and PCPs are all involved in the diagnosis, management and follow-up of AD patients, although differences in regulations may vary across governments (diagnosis and prescriptions are carried out by dementia specialists in some countries). See also practical recommendations.

(2) Before treating cognitive symptoms with ChEIns, clinicians must rule out major contraindications such as sinus bradycardia and AV block.

(3) There is no consensus on the duration of therapy with ChEIns and memantine. We therefore suggest introducing the treatment for 6 months, after which the patient's response should be reviewed. Treatment should be continued if improvement or stabilization is noted on MMSE, IADL and family or caregivers' impression. Treatment should be discontinued if major side effects occur (see table) or if patients significantly deteriorate. However, if patients drastically aggravate after discontinuation, we advise to reintroduce the treatment, in the absence of major contraindications. ChEIns should be continued until a severe stage, when memantine can be introduced. When to stop memantine is not known. We personally suggest discontinuation when the disease is very advanced (MMSE <7) and/or if no benefits are observed, or in the rare case that agitation is noted.

(4) Before treating BPSD, clinicians must particularly rule out delirium (i.e. in agitated patients), try to eliminate environmental triggers (e.g. abnormal light, noise, or a sudden change of nursing staff) and train caregivers and/or nursing staff to recognize side effects in order to prevent increased morbidity or mortality (e.g. falls and bone fractures due to drowsiness or hypotension).

(5) When initiating BPSD treatment, target symptoms (e.g. agitation in the setting of depression or psychosis) should be selected to focus on in the monitoring of the drug treatment.

(6) After initiation of treatment with antidepressants, antipsychotics or antiepileptics, patients should be closely monitored for side effects. Chronic administration should not be the rule and treatment should be as short as possible.

neuronal loss in the main cholinergic nucleus in the forebrain (nucleus basalis of Meynert), is one of the hallmarks of AD [for review, see 3]. This disturbance of the cholinergic system led to development of cholinesterase inhibitors (ChEIns), which enhance cholinergic neurotransmission in the cerebral cortex. Three ChEIns are currently approved in Europe and the US. These have not yet been compared directly in head-to-head trials [4]. Donepezil has few peripheral anticholinesterase activities and is therefore usually well tolerated by patients. Its easy once-daily titration makes it the most popular ChEIn on the market. It has been shown to significantly improve cognition, as assessed with the ADAS-cog, and clinicians' global ratings, for patients with mild to moderate AD compared to a placebo group. It did, however, not improve quality of life measures [5]. Other studies concluded that extended treatment over 6 months is safe and effective in mild to moderate stages [6] as well as in an advanced stage [7]. A nonsponsored trial with patients in similar stages of the disease replicated a small but significant effect of the medication (0.8 point increase in MMSE score compared to placebo), but this result did not delay the need for institutional care of patients [8]. In the same study, a return to baseline cognition level after a six-week placebo washout suggested an absence of disease-modifying activity of the medication. BPSD may be alleviated by donepezil but only modestly [9]. In mild cognitive impairment (MCI), donepezil was the only ChEIn that significantly improved cognitive outcome (MMSE, ADAS-Cog, CDR) after 6 months, but it had no effect on the rate of conversion to AD after 3 years [10].

Galantamine has slightly more gastrointestinal side effects, such as nausea, vomiting, anorexia and weight loss, but these side effects are attenuated in a once-daily prescription. Overall, the clinical efficacy of galantamine is the same as that of donepezil. RCTs demonstrated a significant positive effect of galantamine (16 or 24 mg per day) on cognition and ADL in the treated group over the placebo group [11], and cognitive effects were sustained for up to 36 months [12]. Galantamine, however, has been associated with increased mortality in patients with MCI [13] and is therefore not recommended in this condition.

Rivastigmine is a ChEIn with marked peripheral side effects, and is recommended to be taken with food according to a very slow titration schedule. The advantage of rivastigmine over other cholinesterase inhibitors is that it has an equally high clinical efficacy, but fewer interactions with other medication and less liver metabolism. Although its side effect profile is still a disadvantage [14], a once-daily transdermal patch has recently become available for mild to moderate AD patients. This patch has a much better gastrointestinal profile compared to the oral formulation, and makes rivastigmine as attractive as donepezil and galantamine [15].

Overall, the benefit of ChEIns for patients with AD is a modest improvement in cognition and in ratings on ADL and instrumental ADL (IADL) scales. A severely limiting factor, however, of ChEIns is that only 30–50% of patients respond to the treatment [16]. There is an urgent need for a better identification of the responders, in order to stop treatment in those who do not respond.

In a systematic review, it was concluded that ChEIns offer a small but significant alleviation of BPSD, but its clinical significance remains debatable because most patients presented with mild symptoms only [9], and subsequent studies of rivastigmine and donepezil did not replicate the benefits in patients with severe symptoms [17].

Long-term improvements, such as a significantly reduced rate of nursing home placement or a prolongation of normal ADL and behavior, are still questionable and the results from trials are conflicting [4, 8]. Early studies claimed that ChEIns were cost effective, decreased the need for home care and delayed nursing home placement [18]. However, the only non-sponsored study did not find any nursing home placement benefit in treated patients compared to placebo [8].

Memantine

Memantine is an *N*-methyl-D-aspartate (NMDA) receptor antagonist. NMDA receptors are implicated in learning and memory, and increased NMDA stimulation in AD presumably causes abnormal excitotoxicity in the brain [for review, see 19]. By blocking the increased NMDA stimulation, memantine may have a neuroprotective effect. Twenty mg of memantine daily in two doses significantly stabilizes or even improves cognition and/or IADL, as demonstrated by Reisberg et al. [20] and several other RCTs in patients with moderate to severe AD. There were no more adverse effects in the treatment group than in the placebo group, suggesting a better side effect profile than cholinesterase inhibitors. In current practice, dizziness, confusion and hallucinations are the most frequently reported side effects. A recent meta-analysis of three published studies (two in moderate to severe AD patients and one in mild to moderate AD patients) revealed a significant but very modest benefit of memantine on cognition and global changes [21].

A post-hoc analysis of 6 pooled RCTs showed diminished BPSD in the memantine treatment group compared to the placebo group, particularly for psychosis and agitation/aggression [22]. The same RCTs were included in another analysis, which also demonstrated an improvement of BPSD. This latter study, however, questioned whether there is a clinical benefit of memantine, mainly because of the small effect size [23]. Administration of memantine on a once-daily schedule appeared to be similar to a twice-a-day regimen in terms of efficacy and tolerability [24]. More importantly, a rapid switch from donepezil to memantine was tolerated as well as a stepwise one [25]. This offers a possible practical benefit for patients with side effects or those who deteriorate on ChEIns.

At present, data on the long-term effects of memantine in patients with mild to moderate AD have yet to be reported. There is also still a need for strong evidence of a neuroprotective effect and for reports on side effects in large clinical samples.

Memantine plus Cholinesterase Inhibitors

In one RCT, the combination of memantine and cholinesterase inhibitors was found to be more effective than donepezil alone in AD patients in a moderate to severe stage, in terms of cognition, ADL, global functioning and behavior [26]. However, with results of only one study, there is a lack of consensus about the benefit of this combination, and several medication agencies have not authorized its reimbursement.

Antioxidants

Vitamin E, or α-tocopherol, is an antioxidant agent that was thought to be neuroprotective. One single RCT showed a significant delay in institutionalization, but no effect on other primary or secondary outcomes, including MMSE score [27]. Vitamin E is no longer prescribed for AD.

Ginkgo biloba is derived from a plant with antioxidant properties and has been commercialized in Europe for more than two decades. There have been no large RCTs showing a significant benefit to date, but some results are expected shortly [for a review, see 28]. At present, we do not recommend its use in AD.

Estrogen Replacement

Estrogen replacement therapy has been demonstrated to lead to in vitro cerebral blood flow enhancement, cholinergic neuronal death prevention, and nerve growth factor modulation. Preliminary results of small RCTs were very promising [for review, see 29]. As a consequence, high hopes were placed on this therapy. Unfortunately, large RCTs did not replicate these initial findings, and even showed that estrogen replacement carried with it an increased risk of developing dementia and increased morbidity and mortality rates [30].

Anti-Inflammatory Drugs

Anti-inflammatory drugs – traditional NSAIDs or selective COX-2 inhibitors – also raised high hopes for prevention and treatment of AD, since inflammatory processes (such as activated microglia and cytokine release) have been implicated in AD [for a review, see 31]. Some epidemiologic studies on anti-inflammatory drugs reported a reduced conversion rate to AD. However, several RCTs using COX-2 inhibitors did not show any benefit, or were even suspended due to an increased rate of cardiovascular events [31]. A recent large interventional trial also failed to find any beneficial effects and even showed increased bleeding in the treated group [32]. It is quite possible that anti-inflammatory drugs are ineffective once the AD lesions have become well established, or that the drug has to be administered for a very long period for it to have any measurable effect. We do not currently advocate the use of anti-inflammatory drugs in prevention or treatment of AD.

Vascular Risk Factor Management

Because of the strong relationship between main vascular factors and the amyloid cascade, and because of the aggravating effect of vascular impairments on AD pathology, strict management of high blood pressure, diabetes and cholesterol levels are increasingly recommended, even though meta-analysis with cholesterol-lowering agents [33] and antihypertensive drugs did not show a decrease in the rate of the progression to dementia in patients with respectively high cholesterol and hypertension plus no history of cerebrovascular disease [34]. The lack of an adequately long follow-up period could be one of the reasons for these negative results.

Antipsychotic Agents

Atypical antipsychotic agents have been used generally against symptoms such as agitation, aggression and delusions. They have better extrapyramidal profiles than conventional neuroleptics. However, they have been associated with increased mortality and are still not approved for treatment of AD by federal regulations in most European countries and the USA. Moreover, there have been no trials that have compared the efficacy of different atypical antipsychotic agents. A systematic review including 12 trials plus two additional studies of haloperidol, thioridazine, thioxanthene, chlorpromazine and acetophenazine, did not demonstrate any benefit for patients [9]. Two other systematic reviews concluded that atypical antipsychotics such as clozapine, olanzapine, risperidone and quietapine had only modest efficacy, and one RCT even claimed that these agents (clozapine not included) had no effect on psychosis, aggression or agitation compared to a placebo [35, 36]. They were also found to elicit side effects, including extrapyramidal symptoms and sedation [35]. Increased mortality and stroke risk, although debated due to conflicting results, has been another concern recently [36]. For these reasons, atypical antipsychotic agents should not be routinely used against agitation or psychosis in AD.

Antidepressants

As serotonin neurotransmission is disturbed in both AD and in agitation/aggression and depression [37, 38], many studies have focused on the use of selective serotonin reuptake inhibitors. Several trials have demonstrated that citalopram [39] and sertraline [40] have a beneficial effect in depression in AD. However, because of small sample sizes, insufficient data, absence of significant results and adverse events, a meta-analysis did not support their efficacy and recommended extreme caution [41].

Tricyclic antidepressants such as amitriptyline or nortriptyline should be abandoned because of their anticholinergic side effects, aggravating memory or provoking delirium [42]. Results of RCTs with new antidepressants like venlafaxine, mirtazipine and bupropion have yet to be reported.

Antiepileptic Drugs

There is no evidence that carbamazepine or valproate alleviate BPSD in AD [9], but results of studies with lamotrigine and gabapentin, which are increasingly used in clinical settings, are expected.

RCTs with benzodiazepines in AD have not been carried out, as every clinician is aware of the side effects, such as a decline of memory function, gait disturbances, dependence and possible paradoxical reactions. We suggest benzodiazepines should only be used in the case of brief stressful episodes, with extreme caution and in small doses.

There are no RCT data on buspirone, propranolol, or levecitaretam.

Conclusion

After initial hopes rose with the introduction of cholinesterase inhibitors, new hope comes from a growing understanding of the basic mechanisms causing AD [43]. First, since amyloid peptide plays a central role in AD neuropathology, antiamyloid therapies are thought to slow down or limit progression of the disease. A phase IIa amyloid-beta immunization RCT was interrupted because of meningoencephalitis in 6% of patients, but showed significant clinical benefit in antibody responders [44]. New RCTs with passive and active immunization against amyloid-beta are currently ongoing. Other promising compounds that are anticipated are neuroprotective agents, such as antioxidants and anti-inflammatory agents, which are expected to reduce the damage caused by amyloid proteins. Finally, neurorestorative approaches such as neurotrophic and nerve growth factors, transplantations and stem cell-related interventions are being developed.

Illusions came from various reviews of medications approved in the US and Europe for the treatment of patients with AD. A very recent study concluded that all compounds that have significant positive effects on various measures for cognitive and more global functions, produce little if any clinically meaningful benefits [21]. The same conclusions have been drawn for the effects of atypical antipsychotics on BPSD [35].

There is still a long way to go in the development of treatments. A major challenge is that AD is not a disease in a technical sense, but a complex syndrome exhibiting a diversity of symptoms. We will conclude by giving some specific directions for further research. (1) More fundamental research is necessary to allow for an earlier and more accurate diagnosis and follow-up of the progression of the disease (e.g. by identifying better biomarkers). This could prevent unnecessary neuronal damage and block amyloid deposition and neurofibrillary tangle formation. (2) More non-sponsored or independent RCTs should be carried out. (3) Head-to-head trials are needed, which compare the different medications that are currently available (e.g. the three available ChEIns; ChEIns and memantine; the different antidepressants; atypical and classical antipsychotics; antiepileptics). (4) We also need to reassess our clinical scales, to ensure accurate clinical monitoring of patients under treatment of current symptomatic agents, or of possible future disease-modifying agents. Sensitive clinical scales are particularly important in this latter case, because the most likely candidates to be treated with future disease-modifying agents are early AD patients in whom the decline is slow, and clinical changes are variable and subtle. The use of sensitive clinical scales would require less lengthy and therefore less expensive trials, and would make sponsoring by industries more likely. (5) Furthermore, there is an urgent need for clinical markers that are sensitive, widely available, and cost effective. Dual-task-related gait change could be an interesting candidate, since gait and cognition are closely linked. Moreover, a recent open-labeled pilot study demonstrated an alteration of gait parameters in patients with AD, treated with galantamine [45]. (6) More appropriate start and termination points of medication need to be identified, to prevent unnecessary treatment when no efficacy is proven. (7) We also need to better explain medication-related issues (i.e. the precise benefits that can be expected) to our patients and their families. (8) Finally, better recognition and integration of the cognitive decline and BPSD is needed, and we have to start to develop additional nonpharmacological therapies.

All these above-mentioned strategies may contribute to improve patient care and reduce the emotional and financial burden on families and governments.

References

1 McKhann G, Drachman D, Folstein M, Katzman R, Price D, Stadlan EM: Clinical diagnosis of Alzheimer's disease: report of the NINCDS-ADRDA Work Group under the auspices of Department of Health and Human Services Task Force on Alzheimer's Disease. Neurology 1984;34:939–944.

2 Assal F, Cummings JL: Neuropsychiatric symptoms in the dementias. Curr Opin Neurol 2002;15:445–450.

3 Whitehouse PJ, Price DL, Clark AW, Coyle JT, DeLong MR: Alzheimer disease: evidence for selective loss of cholinergic neurons in the nucleus basalis. Ann Neurol 1981;10:122–126.

4 Trinh NH, Hoblyn J, Mohanty S, Yaffe K: Efficacy of cholinesterase inhibitors in the treatment of neuropsychiatric symptoms and functional impairment in Alzheimer disease: a meta-analysis. J Am Med Assoc 2003; 289:210–216.

5 Rogers SL, Farlow MR, Doody RS, Mohs R, Friedhoff LT: A 24-week, double-blind, placebo-controlled trial of donepezil in patients with Alzheimer's disease. Donepezil Study Group. Neurology 1998;50:136–145.

6 Winblad B, Engedal K, Soininen H, Verhey F, Waldemar G, Wimo A, Wetterholm AL, Zhang R, Haglund A, Subbiah P: A 1-year, randomized, placebo-controlled study of donepezil in patients with mild to moderate AD. Neurology 2001;57:489–495.

7 Winblad B, Kilander L, Eriksson S, Minthon L, Batsman S, Wetterholm AL, Jansson-Blixt C, Haglund A: Donepezil in patients with severe Alzheimer's disease: double-blind, parallel-group, placebo-controlled study. Lancet 2006;367:1057–1065.

8 Courtney C, Farrell D, Gray R, Hills R, Lynch L, Sellwood E, Edwards S, Hardyman W, Raftery J, Crome P, Lendon C, Shaw H, Bentham P: Long-term donepezil treatment in 565 patients with Alzheimer's disease (AD2000): randomised double-blind trial. Lancet 2004;363:2105–2115.

9 Sink KM, Holden KF, Yaffe K: Pharmacological treatment of neuropsychiatric symptoms of dementia: a review of the evidence. J Am Med Assoc 2005;293:596–608.

10 Petersen RC, Thomas RG, Grundman M, Bennett D, Doody R, Ferris S, Galasko D, Jin S, Kaye J, Levey A, Pfeiffer E, Sano M, van Dyck CH, Thal LJ: Vitamin E and donepezil for the treatment of mild cognitive impairment. N Engl J Med 2005;352:2379–2388.

11 Wilcock GK, Lilienfeld S, Gaens E: Efficacy and safety of galantamine in patients with mild to moderate Alzheimer's disease: multicentre randomised controlled trial. Galantamine International-1 Study Group. Br Med J 2000;321:1445–1449.

12 Raskind MA, Peskind ER, Truyen L, Kershaw P, Damaraju CV: The cognitive benefits of galantamine are sustained for at least 36 months: a long-term extension trial. Arch Neurol 2004;61:252–256.

13 Mayor S: Regulatory authorities review use of galantamine in mild cognitive impairment. Br Med J 2005;330: 276.

14 Rosler M, Anand R, Cicin-Sain A, Gauthier S, Agid Y, Dal-Bianco P, Stahelin HB, Hartman R, Gharabawi M: Efficacy and safety of rivastigmine in patients with Alzheimer's disease: international randomised controlled trial. Br Med J 1999;318:633–638.

15 Winblad B, Grossberg G, Frolich L, Farlow M, Zechner S, Nagel J, Lane R: IDEAL: a 6-month, double-blind, placebo-controlled study of the first skin patch for Alzheimer disease. Neurology 2007;69: S14–S22.

16 Cummings JL: Use of cholinesterase inhibitors in clinical practice: evidence-based recommendations. Am J Geriatr Psychiatry 2003;11:131–145.

17 Howard RJ, Juszczak E, Ballard CG, Bentham P, Brown RG, Bullock R, Burns AS, Holmes C, Jacoby R, Johnson T, Knapp M, Lindesay J, O'Brien JT, Wilcock G, Katona C, Jones RW, DeCesare J, Rodger M: Donepezil for the treatment of agitation in Alzheimer's disease. N Engl J Med 2007;357:1382–1392.

18 Neumann PJ, Hermann RC, Kuntz KM, Araki SS, Duff SB, Leon J, Berenbaum PA, Goldman PA, Williams LW, Weinstein MC: Cost-effectiveness of donepezil in the treatment of mild or moderate Alzheimer's disease. Neurology 1999;52:1138–1145.

19 Parsons CG, Danysz W, Quack G: Memantine is a clinically well tolerated N-methyl-D-aspartate (NMDA) receptor antagonist – a review of preclinical data. Neuropharmacology 1999;38:735–767.

20 Reisberg B, Doody R, Stoffler A, Schmitt F, Ferris S, Mobius HJ: Memantine in moderate-to-severe Alzheimer's disease. N Engl J Med 2003;348:1333–1341.

21 Qaseem A, Snow V, Cross JT Jr, Forciea MA, Hopkins R Jr, Shekelle P, Adelman A, Mehr D, Schellhase K, Campos-Outcalt D, Santaguida P, Owens DK: Current pharmacologic treatment of dementia: a clinical practice guideline from the American College of Physicians and the American Academy of Family Physicians. Ann Intern Med 2008;148:370–378.

22 Gauthier S, Loft H, Cummings J: Improvement in behavioural symptoms in patients with moderate to severe Alzheimer's disease by memantine: a pooled data analysis. Int J Geriatr Psychiatry 2008;23:537–545.

23 Maidment ID, Fox CG, Boustani M, Rodriguez J, Brown RC, Katona CL: Efficacy of memantine on behavioral and psychological symptoms related to dementia: a systematic meta-analysis. Ann Pharmacother 2008;42:32–38.

24 Jones RW, Bayer A, Inglis F, Barker A, Phul R: Safety and tolerability of once-daily versus twice-daily memantine: a randomised, double-blind study in moderate to severe Alzheimer's disease. Int J Geriatr Psychiatry 2007;22:258–262.

25 Waldemar G, Hyvarinen M, Josiassen MK, Korner A, Lehto H, Wetterberg P: Tolerability of switching from donepezil to memantine treatment in patients with moderate to severe Alzheimer's disease. Int J Geriatr Psychiatry 2008;23:979–981.

26 Tariot PN, Farlow MR, Grossberg GT, Graham SM, McDonald S, Gergel I: Memantine treatment in patients with moderate to severe Alzheimer disease already receiving donepezil: a randomized controlled trial. J Am Med Assoc 2004;291:317–324.

27 Sano M, Ernesto C, Thomas RG, Klauber MR, Schafer K, Grundman M, Woodbury P, Growdon J, Cotman CW, Pfeiffer E, Schneider LS, Thal LJ: A controlled trial of selegiline, alpha-tocopherol, or both as treatment for Alzheimer's disease. The Alzheimer's Disease Cooperative Study. N Engl J Med 1997;336:1216–1222.

28 Ramassamy C, Longpre F, Christen Y: Ginkgo biloba extract (EGb 761) in Alzheimer's disease: is there any evidence? Curr Alzheimer Res 2007;4:253–262.

29 Henderson VW: Estrogen-containing hormone therapy and Alzheimer's disease risk: understanding discrepant inferences from observational and experimental research. Neuroscience 2006;138: 1031–1039.
30 Rapp SR, Espeland MA, Shumaker SA, Henderson VW, Brunner RL, Manson JE, Gass ML, Stefanick ML, Lane DS, Hays J, Johnson KC, Coker LH, Dailey M, Bowen D: Effect of estrogen plus progestin on global cognitive function in postmenopausal women: the Women's Health Initiative Memory Study: a randomized controlled trial. J Am Med Assoc 2003; 289:2663–2672.
31 McGeer PL, McGeer EG: NSAIDs and Alzheimer disease: epidemiological, animal model and clinical studies. Neurobiol Aging 2007;28:639–647.
32 Bentham P, Gray R, Sellwood E, Hills R, Crome P, Raftery J: Aspirin in Alzheimer's disease (AD2000): a randomised open-label trial. Lancet Neurol 2008; 7:41–49.
33 Zhou B, Teramukai S, Fukushima M: Prevention and treatment of dementia or Alzheimer's disease by statins: a meta-analysis. Dement Geriatr Cogn Disord 2007;23:194–201.
34 McGuinness B, Todd S, Passmore P, Bullock R: The effects of blood pressure lowering on development of cognitive impairment and dementia in patients without apparent prior cerebrovascular disease. Cochrane Database Syst Rev 2006:CD004034.
35 Schneider LS, Tariot PN, Dagerman KS, Davis SM, Hsiao JK, Ismail MS, Lebowitz BD, Lyketsos CG, Ryan JM, Stroup TS, Sultzer DL, Weintraub D, Lieberman JA: Effectiveness of atypical antipsychotic drugs in patients with Alzheimer's disease. N Engl J Med 2006;355:1525–1538.
36 Schneider LS, Dagerman KS, Insel P: Risk of death with atypical antipsychotic drug treatment for dementia: meta-analysis of randomized placebo-controlled trials. J Am Med Assoc 2005;294: 1934–1943.
37 Assal F, Alarcon M, Solomon EC, Masterman D, Geschwind DH, Cummings JL: Association of the serotonin transporter and receptor gene polymorphisms in neuropsychiatric symptoms in Alzheimer disease. Arch Neurol 2004;61:1249–1253.
38 Assal F, Cummings JL: Neuropathological changes underlying neuropsychiatric symptoms on Alzheimer's disease; in Gauthier S, Cummings JL (eds): Alzheimer's Disease and Related Disorders Annual 2002. London, Martin Dunitz, 2002, pp 199–215.
39 Nyth AL, Gottfries CG: The clinical efficacy of citalopram in treatment of emotional disturbances in dementia disorders. A Nordic multicentre study. Br J Psychiatry 1990;157:894–901.
40 Lyketsos CG, Sheppard JM, Steele CD, Kopunek S, Steinberg M, Baker AS, Brandt J, Rabins PV: Randomized, placebo-controlled, double-blind clinical trial of sertraline in the treatment of depression complicating Alzheimer's disease: initial results from the Depression in Alzheimer's Disease study. Am J Psychiatry 2000;157:1686–1689.
41 Bains J, Birks JS, Dening TR: The efficacy of antidepressants in the treatment of depression in dementia. Cochrane Database Syst Rev 2002:CD003944.
42 Taragano FE, Lyketsos CG, Mangone CA, Allegri RF, Comesana-Diaz E: A double-blind, randomized, fixed-dose trial of fluoxetine vs. amitriptyline in the treatment of major depression complicating Alzheimer's disease. Psychosomatics 1997;38:246–252.
43 Cummings JL, Doody R, Clark C: Disease-modifying therapies for Alzheimer disease: challenges to early intervention. Neurology 2007;69: 1622–1634.
44 Gilman S, Koller M, Black RS, Jenkins L, Griffith SG, Fox NC, Eisner L, Kirby L, Rovira MB, Forette F, Orgogozo JM: Clinical effects of Abeta immunization (AN1792) in patients with AD in an interrupted trial. Neurology 2005;64:1553–1562.
45 Assal F, Allali G, Kressig RW, Herrmann FR, Beauchet O: Galantamine improves gait performance in patients with Alzheimer's disease. J Am Geriatr Soc 2008;56:946–947.

Frédéric Assal, MD
Faculty of Medicine and Neurology, Department of Clinical Neurosciences
University Hospitals of Geneva, rue du Micheli-du-Crest 24
CH–1211 Geneva (Switzerland)
Tel. +41 22 372 83 18, Fax +41 22 372 83 32, E-Mail frederic.assal@hcuge.ch

Giannakopoulos P, Hof PR (eds): Dementia in Clinical Practice.
Front Neurol Neurosci. Basel, Karger, 2009, vol 24, pp 66–78

Investigations in Primary Care

Anna Poggesi · Leonardo Pantoni

Department of Neurological and Psychiatric Sciences, University of Florence, Florence, Italy

Abstract

Vascular cognitive impairment relates to subjects who have a broad spectrum of cognitive deficits, including all forms of mild to severe cognitive impairment associated with and presumed to be caused by cerebrovascular diseases. The latter may be represented by multiple cortical infarcts, multiple subcortical infarcts, or both, silent infarcts, strategic infarcts, small-vessel disease with white matter lesions, and lacunes, all more or less related to stroke. Some authors also include in the category of vascular cognitive impairment Alzheimer's disease patients with evidence of additional vascular lesions. The recognition of early cognitive decline in the primary care setting is an important step as it may allow an early referral of patients to the specialist level, thus permitting a correct diagnosis of the etiologic subtype and the best treatment approach for that particular patient. The aim of this chapter is to provide an overview of the role of the primary care physician in the screening of patients with suspected vascular cognitive decline. Patients in whom screening for cognitive decline could be of clinical relevance are depicted, and a brief overview of investigations and diagnostic tests in the primary care setting is outlined. This specific diagnostic approach includes suggestions on how to take the clinical history, how to perform the physical examination, and on how to choose the appropriate tools for the cognitive and non-cognitive screening; finally, the role of neuroimaging in the primary care setting is illustrated.

Dementia is defined as a significant loss of intellectual abilities such as memory, attention, orientation, judgment, language, motor and spatial skills, severe enough to interfere with social or occupational functioning [1]. Dementia is labeled as 'vascular' when it is believed that the syndrome is caused by cerebrovascular diseases. The concept of vascular dementia (VaD) has undergone substantial re-evaluation over the last years, and both terms 'vascular' and 'dementia' have been criticized by some authors [2]. One of the main concerns is that VaD is a heterogeneous group of diseases rather than a unique pathological process, with different causes and a broader spectrum of cognitive impairment, with only part of the patients being definable as overtly demented [2]. Given the complexity of the relationship between cerebrovascular diseases and cognition, a broader concept, vascular cognitive impairment (VCI) was thus introduced some years ago in order to include all the possible aspects of this complex relation [3, 4]. VCI refers to all forms of mild to severe cognitive impairment associated with and presumed to be caused by cerebrovascular diseases [4]. This term, therefore, includes VCI without dementia as well as VaD. The concept of VCI covers subjects who have cognitive impairment related to stroke, multiple cortical infarcts, multiple subcortical infarcts, or both, silent infarcts, strategic infarcts, small-vessel disease with white matter lesions, and lacunes. Some authors also include in the category of VCI Alzheimer's disease (AD) patients who also have evidence of vascular lesions [5].

The aim of the present chapter is to provide an overview of the possible role of the primary care physician in the screening of patients with suspected VaD and VCI. Since data available on this topic are limited, most of our writing is a proposal for the role of primary care physicians in this setting derived from our experience in the field, representing our beliefs of what the role of our primary care colleagues should be in this sense.

Role of the Primary Care Physician in Screening for Vascular Dementia and Cognitive Impairment

It is probably not a clinical challenge to diagnose dementia when the symptoms are of moderate to severe degree. Differently, it may be more challenging to detect the degrees of cognitive impairment that precedes dementia onset, so called mild cognitive impairment [6]. The recognition of early cognitive decline in the primary care setting is an important step as it may allow an early referral of patients to the specialist levels, thus permitting a correct diagnosis of the subtype and the best treatment approach for that particular patient.

Target Populations

In our view, in the field of VaD and VCI, primary care physician may face generally three types of patients in whom screening for cognitive decline may be of clinical relevance, and thus recommended: (1) patients with vascular risk factors; (2) patients with subjective or minimally cognitive or behavioral disturbances as referred by a next of kin; (3) patients who returned home after a stroke.

Patients with Vascular Risk Factors

Patients with vascular risk factors are at increasing risk of developing cognitive impairment during their lives. According to Hachinski and Bowler [3], these patients are in a 'brain at risk' stage. The link between vascular risk factors and cognitive decline is in some cases related to the occurrence of major cerebrovascular events, while in other instances vascular risk factors lead to a progressive development of initially silent

Table 1. Major risk factors for VCI and VaD distinguished as risk factors directly related to VCI, risk factors for stroke (as a determinant of VCI) and risk factors common to atherosclerosis and AD

Risk factors directly related to VCI [adapted from 9]	Risk factors for stroke as a determinant of VCI [adapted from 11, 12]	Risk factors common to atherosclerosis and AD [adapted from 9, 13]
Age	Age	Age
Hypertension	Hypertension	Hypertension
Diabetes mellitus	Diabetes mellitus	Diabetes mellitus
Hyperlipidemia	Hyperlipidemia	Hyperlipidemia
Cigarette smoking	Cigarette smoking	Cigarette smoking
Alcohol consumption	Alcohol consumption	Hyperhomocysteinemia
Obesity	Obesity	Obesity
Physical inactivity	Physical inactivity	Metabolic syndrome
Metabolic syndrome	Metabolic syndrome	ApoE ε4 polymorphism
Hyperhomocysteinemia	Carotid stenosis	Systemic inflammation
Stroke	Atrial fibrillation	Hormone replacement therapy
Stroke related features:	Ischemic heart disease	
– Volume of cerebral vascular lesions	Valvular heart disease	
	Psychosocial stress	
– Location of cerebral vascular lesions	Diet (low fruit and vegetables intake)	
– Number of cerebral vascular lesions	Hyperhomocysteinemia	
	Hormone replacement therapy	
– White matter lesions		
– Silent cerebral infarcts		

vascular changes in the brain that eventually cause cognitive decline. Some vascular risk factors are also thought to be associated with AD type pathology [7, 8].

Table 1 reports the major risk factors for vascular cognitive decline and dementia; these have been divided into factors directly related to the cognitive decline, factors related to stroke (as a determinant of cognitive decline) or factors common to atherosclerosis and AD. Only a few studies have evaluated the effect of risk factors for stroke on the probability of developing cognitive decline before the actual occurrence of stroke, corroborating the intuitive conclusion that subjects at increased risk for stroke are also at increased risk for dementia [9, 10]. Moreover, from large epidemiological studies we have learned that VaD and AD share with stroke a number of vascular risk factors. For some of these risk factors, a large body of evidence is available showing a relation with cognitive decline, for others this relationship may be realistically inferred for example from their association with stroke.

Among the modifiable risk factors, certainly arterial hypertension has a major role. The relationship between blood pressure and cognitive function and dementia has, in recent years, received much attention from epidemiological research. From one recent review, it clearly came out that there exists a discrepancy between results of cross-sectional studies and longitudinal studies addressing this issue [14]. In fact, cross-sectional studies have shown an inverse association between blood pressure and the prevalence of dementia, whereas longitudinal studies yield mixed results that largely depend on the age at which blood pressure is measured and the time interval between blood pressure and outcome assessments. Evidence suggests that both high and low blood pressures play a part in the development and progression of cognitive impairment and dementia, depending on age [14]. A second group of patients at risk of developing cognitive decline are diabetics. A large body of evidence is emerging suggesting a close relationship between diabetes mellitus and the increased risk of both VaD and AD, with various pathological changes contributing to the dementia process [15, 16].

Searching for VCI in all the patients with at least one of the risk factors listed in table 1 is likely beyond the possibility of each primary care physician. However, we believe it is important at any level to draw the attention to these groups of patients as possible candidates to cognitive decline because this is the stage when much can be done to prevent this poor outcome.

Patients with Subjective or Minimal Cognitive or Behavioral Disturbances

Subjective memory complaints are frequently reported by healthy elderly persons [17]. Some community-based studies suggest that 35–40% of healthy, nondemented elderly persons above the age of 75 years report problems with memory [18]. Such memory complaints may be 'benign', when unrelated to brain pathological processes and not associated with decline of functional performances.

Few studies have examined longitudinally individuals with self-reported memory complaints, and results appear discordant. Some have found that subjective memory loss is associated with an increased risk of developing dementia [19–21], while others have found that subjective memory complaints do not correlate with memory problems and may correlate better with depressive symptoms or personality traits [22, 23]. Thus, it is difficult to know when memory complaints precede dementia or instead are simply manifestations of aging or other conditions such as depression [23]. In general, patients' complaints should not be ignored, as in the mild stages of dementia these subjects often have some insight into their own deficit.

Family members, or close friends (informants) often detect memory loss before the patient. Corroborating information from an informant is helpful, and informant questionnaires are considered as effective as brief cognitive tests at screening for dementia [24]. In fact, it has been demonstrated that informants' reports may predict the development of dementia in patients who currently have normal test results [23]. Although not all informants are equally helpful, with spouses or others who live with the patient giving the most accurate assessment of cognitive status [25], many older adults do not have reliable and knowledgeable informants, making a direct evaluation of the subject more important. Concerns regarding memory, changes in personality or behavior, or the performance in daily activities, whether expressed by the patient or an informant, should trigger an evaluation for both dementing illnesses and mood disorders [26]. If a clinician has concerns about a patient's cognitive status, cognitive testing to the patient could be combined with questionnaires to a reliable informant to improve accuracy in the diagnosis [27, 28].

Patients Who Returned Home after a Stroke

The term poststroke dementia has been coined to indicate all dementia syndromes occurring in close time relation with a stroke. In fact, stroke increases considerably the risk of dementia, with prevalence rates ranging from 13.6 to 32% 3 months to 1 year after stroke, and incidence rates of new-onset dementia after stroke ranging from 24% within 3 years to 33.3% within 5 years [29]. Despite improvement in stroke prevention and treatment, the prevalence of poststroke dementia is likely to increase in the future because of increased survival after stroke and ageing of the population [30]. Patients with poststroke dementia have higher mortality rates and are more often functionally impaired [29]. The detection of cognitive decline after stroke may have relevant consequences in terms of management of patients, better appreciation of outcome, prevision of drug therapy compliance, and prognostic information for family burden. A recent review outlined some aspects of neuropsychological functioning, such as presence of neglect, aphasia, anosognosia, verbal memory and attention deficits to be good predictors of post-stroke functional outcomes, thus suggesting that these areas of neuropsychological functioning could be targeted for rehabilitative efforts [31]. Ideally, screening for cognitive decline should be initiated in the acute stroke unit setting; however, not all stroke patients are admitted to stroke units, and a number of obstacles may delay the screening for cognitive decline after stroke: in this case, the task may eventually rely on the assessment of the primary care physician.

Taking the Clinical History

The collection of information about the clinical history may be very relevant for the appreciation of dementia subtypes. AD is a well-characterized syndrome where the onset, progression, clinical and neuropsychological features are well defined and usually typical. In contrast, VaD is characterized by a wide variety of clinical and neuropsychological features mostly depending on the different pathological processes underlying the dementia syndrome. In AD, the onset is usually gradual, the progression is a constant and insidious decline and there is an early impairment in memory function. In VaD, all these clinical characteristics depend on the type of processes subsiding the cognitive problem. The onset may be gradual when the main pathological processes are white matter lesions, or may be sudden when it follows a stroke (ischemic or hemorrhagic); in the latter case, both the presence of multiple infarcts or the location of a single one (strategic) may be responsible for the clinical picture. Cognitive deterioration may be very slow, when depending on white matter lesions and their progression or with the classical stepwise or fluctuating course due to the multiple stroke events [32].

Cognitive Screening for Dementia

Neuropsychological assessment remains of fundamental importance in the diagnosis of dementia as it documents a significant cognitive decline and may reveal specific patterns of cognitive dysfunction, hinting at the cause of the dementia [33]. The pattern of cognitive deficits in VaD and VCI may be one that includes all cognitive domains, but there is usually a preponderance of so-called 'executive' dysfunction, defined as the impairment in cognitive skills that are responsible for the planning, initiation, sequencing, and monitoring of complex goal-directed behavior [34]. Carrying out the neuropsychological assessment at an early stage of dementia has the advantage to characterize and assess the cognitive and noncognitive functions; these data can then be integrated with other clinical aspects into a broader syndrome [35].

Patients can be evaluated with structured or semi-structured interviews and with neuropsychological test batteries. Many instruments exist for evaluating a patient with suspected cognitive impairment. For many reasons, including time-constrained general medical appointments, the subtlety of early impairment, and the poor sensitivity of many brief screening instruments, no single instrument is ideal for all settings [26]. Recently, the development of harmonization standards for the diagnosis and assessment of patients with early stage of VCI in clinical and research setting has been carried out in a collaborative effort [36]. This consensus has produced a proposal for neuropsychological assessment to be both sensitive to a wide range of abilities and particularly aimed to assess executive functions. The Neuropsychological Working Group has assembled 3 separate protocols: (1) a 60-min protocol, containing tests for the assessment of four domains (executive/activation, language, visuospatial, and memory) plus tests for neurobehavioral changes and mood; (2) a 30-min protocol in which tests were selected from the previous level to be used as a clinical screening instrument for patients with suspected VCI; (3) a 5-min protocol as a quick screening tool in the office of primary care physicians [36]. This last consisted of selected subtests from the Montreal Cognitive Assessment including a 5-word immediate and delayed memory test, a 6-item orientation task and a one-letter phonemic fluency test (the letter F). When more time is available, some other parts of the Montreal Cognitive Assessment could be used such as a cube and a clock drawing task with a simple scoring routine, a 3-item picture naming task, a short 'Trails B' paradigm and other brief attention, language and abstraction tasks. The use of Mini-Mental State Examination [37] was rejected mainly because of its low sensitivity for proving executive dysfunctions [36].

As the authors of this workshop have correctly pointed out, the published recommendations represent the 'beginning' rather than the 'end'. In fact, most of the available literature addressing the issue of different strategies for the detection of dementia in the primary care setting deals with AD. Thus, this has to be considered the first attempt to create new and dedicated instruments for VCI and VaD. While the final diagnosis of VCI and VaD probably cannot rely entirely on only the primary physician's efforts, the proposed brief screening battery can likely help in the selection of patients taken from the 3 above described settings and in referring the patient to the specialist.

Screening for Noncognitive Disturbances

Functional Performance

Impairment in activities of daily living due to cognitive decline is an essential part of the criteria for dementia and should always be assessed in the diagnostic workup. This decline in every day functional abilities has a great influence on the quality of life of patients and their families. Assessment of function in daily living should thus be part of the diagnostic process as a first step in order to distinguish a mild cognitive impairment where functionality is preserved from dementia, and in the long term to evaluate the need for personal and institutional care. The two classical fields measured are: basic activities of daily living (activities that are important for self-care such as dressing, hygiene, continence, and eating) and instrumental activities of daily living (activities that are important for maintenance in a specific environment such as meal preparation, telephoning, housework, taking care of finance and correspondence, going on an outing, taking medications, and so on). Different scales are available and used to objectively measure these abilities in dementia, although most of them were designed to assess functional decline in AD patients. These scales can be administered to both the patient and the caregiver, the latter being probably the best choice for obtaining more reliable information.

Widely used scales include the Activities of Daily Living (ADL) Scale [38], the Instrumental Activities of Daily Living (IADL) Scale [39], and the Disability Assessment for Dementia Scale [40]. Other scales recommended by the European Federation of Neurological Societies Guidelines for the Diagnosis and Management of Alzheimer's Disease [41] are the Alzheimer Disease Cooperative Study ADL Scale [42], the Functional Activities Questionnaire [43], and the Progressive Deterioration Scale [44]. The administration of ADL and IADL scales appears particularly suited for the primary care physician's setting.

Mood and Behavioral Screening

Noncognitive psychiatric and behavioral disturbances are common features of dementia. These include apathy, disinhibition, agitation/aggression, depression, psychosis, appetite changes, and sleep disturbances. Although, these disturbances vary according to the severity of dementia, they might also signal the onset of the disease and often fluctuate and recur. These symptoms are associated with a more rapid cognitive and functional decline, and often lead to caregivers' stress and are among the main reasons for institutionalization [45]. In a recent review, neuropsychiatric manifestations were found to be very common in mild cognitive impairment, occurring in 35–75% of patients, the most common being depression, apathy, anxiety, and irritability [46]. These data suggest that certain neuropsychiatric features could serve as clinical indicators of future conversion to dementia, particularly AD [46]. Studies of the neuropsychiatric disturbances in patients with VaD are few and the results are controversial. Noncognitive psychiatric and behavioral disturbances are thought to vary according to dementia subtypes, thus contributing to the differential diagnosis of the different dementia subtypes. One study has demonstrated that, compared to AD, patients with VaD had higher frequency of decreased affect and withdrawal, and more severe psychomotor slowing, thus confirming the original hypothesis that depression and apathy are more related to VaD [47]. Other recent studies confirmed that behavioral disturbances were very common in patients with dementia, regardless of the dementia type, and found only minor differences in the prevalence and types of behavioral disturbances between AD and VaD patients [48, 49].

Despite these controversial findings, it is of utmost importance to perform a screening of mood and behavior in patients with suspected VCI. Several rating instruments have been designed for this purpose, enquiring not only about the presence or absence of different symptoms, but also about their frequency, severity and impact on the caregiver; repeated use of such scales can also be useful in monitoring the effects of treatment interventions. The scales should be administered to a close family member or to the caregiver. Different screening tools are available for the detection of these noncognitive disturbances, and among these the Neuropsychiatric Inventory is considered a standard tool. It assesses 10 behavioral disturbances occurring in dementia patients: delusions, hallucinations, dysphoria, anxiety, agitation/aggression, euphoria, disinhibition, irritability/lability, apathy, and aberrant motor activity [50]. Other suitable scales are the BEHAVE-AD [51], and the Manchester and Oxford Universities Scale for the Psychopathological Assessment of Dementia [52]. However, it should be noted that these scales are quite complex and require extended time for administration which makes them unsuitable tools for the primary care physician setting.

Physical Examination

Patients with suspected or clear VCI should undergo a physical examination particularly focusing on the cardiovascular system. Peripheral pulses should be assessed, blood pressure and heart rhythm should be checked and recorded, thoracic and carotid auscultation should be performed. Height and weight should be recorded, and body mass index calculated. Also, waist circumference should be determined.

The neurological examination has a specific role in the field of VaD, and attempts to formalize it have been proposed in the past. The Hachinski Ischemic Score was proposed more than 30 years ago as an instrument capable of differentiating multi-infarct dementia from AD [53]. The general features of the scale included abrupt onset, prior history of stroke, stepwise deterioration, somatic complaints, emotional lability, history of hypertension, and focal neurological signs and symptoms. These latter are in fact considered as characteristic features of VaD, capable of distinguishing this latter from neurodegenerative forms, and different clinical criteria include them as a proof of cerebrovascular contribution to dementia. However, little is known about the prevalence of specific neurological signs in the different subtypes of VaD. From one recent study of a large sample of VaD patients, it came out that the specific neurological signs demonstrated by patients with VaD were different according to the type of vascular lesions evidenced by neuroimaging. Subtle signs, including dysarthria and extrapyramidal signs were more prevalent among patients with small vessel disease, while lateralized sensorimotor changes and aphasia were more related to large vessel disease [54]. Also a difference in gait pattern between small vessel and large vessel VaD patients was found, with a hemiplegic type gait disturbance in large vessel disease and a parkinsonian type gait disturbance in small vessel disease [54].

Neuroimaging

Nowadays, neuroimaging is one of the most important investigations in the workup of dementia to aid in the differential diagnosis and management decisions. Traditionally, imaging is important as a means to exclude treatable causes of cognitive decline, and in practice parameter on the diagnosis of dementia, structural neuroimaging, either computed tomography (CT) or magnetic resonance imaging (MRI), is recommended as a guideline in the routine initial evaluation of these patients [41, 55]. Structural neuroimaging should be performed in order to exclude those conditions that are potentially amenable to (usually surgical) treatment, such as neoplasms, hematoma, or hydrocephalus, although these potentially reversible conditions underlie only 1–10% of all dementias [56, 57].

Neuroimaging in general, and MRI in particular, is increasingly regarded as a mandatory part of the investigation of patients with suspected dementia as it can add positive or negative value in the differential diagnosis of the more common types of dementias. According to the consensus criteria [58], absence of vascular lesions on brain MRI rules out a diagnosis of VaD; however, there are no pathognomonic brain CT or MR images of VaD [59]. Thus, correlation with the clinical evidence is mandatory. MRI plays a major role in detecting the type of vascular pathology possibly responsible for the cognitive decline in a particular patient. Imaging evidence of vascular pathology includes 'large vessel' (large territorial or strategic infarcts) and 'small vessel' disease (lacunes and white matter hyperintensities). Neuroimaging also represents one of the most important elements to distinguish AD from VaD.

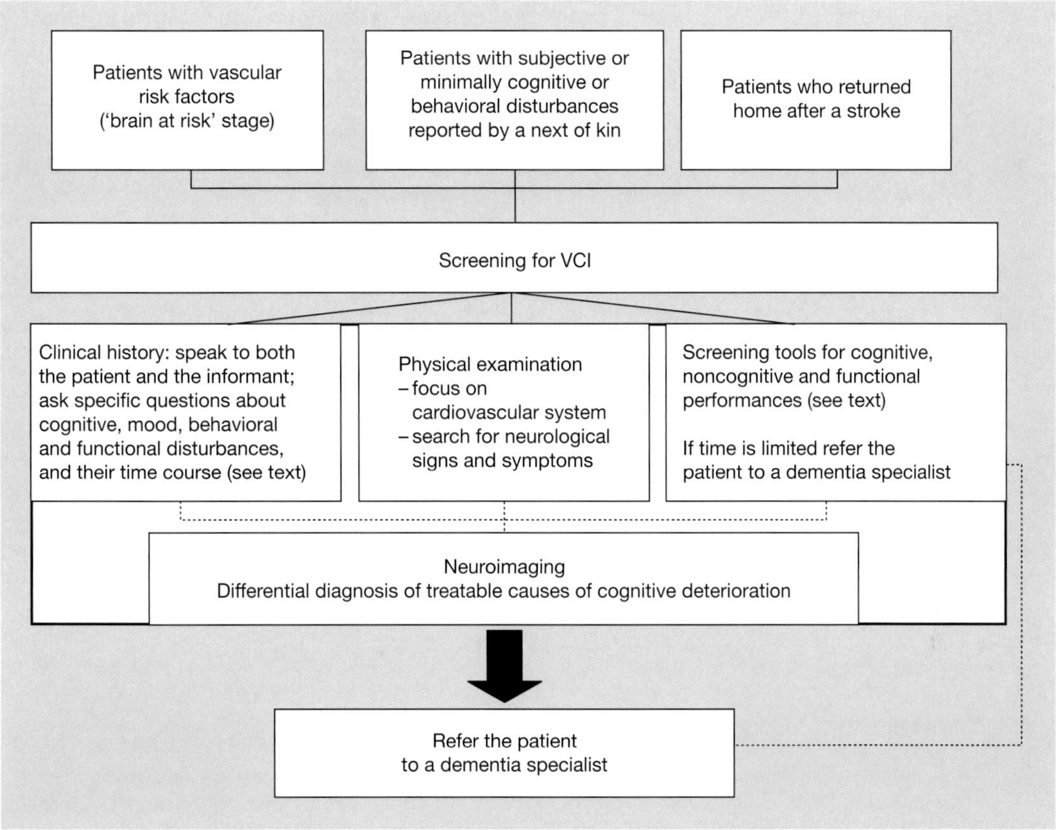

Fig. 1. Proposed algorithm for primary care physicians in the screening for VCI.

We believe that the full appreciation of neuroimaging features applies more to dementia specialists rather than to primary care physicians; however, a first-line imaging evaluation (for example with CT scan) should likely be carried out before sending the patients to the specialist, especially because it may guide the referral to the proper one.

Concluding Remarks

Nowadays, the detection of cognitive impairment at an early stage has become widely proposed, particularly in primary care setting [60]. Previous guidelines in 1996 did not find evidence to advise for or against screening for dementia, the most important problem with the evidence for screening for dementia being the uncertainty of the effectiveness of treatment. However, it should be noted that most of the available data derive from research in the field of AD, while little has been done so far for what concerns VaD and VCI. Available knowledge on risk factors suggests that these conditions could benefit from preventive strategies and the improved control of modifiable risk factors more than degenerative forms. Effective screening, apart form allowing an early referral of patients to the specialist levels, permitting a correct diagnosis of the dementia subtype and the best treatment approach for that particular patient, also gives the opportunity to patients and their families to plan and organize important issues such as health care, safety, and finances.

In the field of VaD and VCI, we identified three types of patients in whom screening for cognitive decline could be of clinical relevance: (1) patients with vascular risk factors; (2) patients with subjective or minimally cognitive or behavioral disturbances as reported by a next of kin; (3) patients who returned home after a stroke. Suggestions for investigations and diagnostic approach have been outlined and are summarized in figure 1. It is worthy to underline the fact that most of the available literature on screening instruments suggested for primary care is related to the AD type of dementia, while little has been done so far in the field of VaD. The first attempt to develop standard tools for the diagnosis and assessment of patients with early stage of VCI in clinical and research setting has recently been completed in a multinational effort [36].

References

1 American Psychiatric Association: Diagnostic and Statistical Manual of Mental Disorders, ed 4. Washington, American Psychiatric Association, 1994.

2 Pantoni L: Subtypes of vascular dementia and their pathogenesis: a critical overview; in Bowler J, Hachinski V (eds): Vascular Cognitive Impairment: Preventable Dementia. Oxford, Oxford University Press, 2003, pp 217–229.

3 Hachinski VC, Bowler JV: Vascular dementia. Neurology 1993;43:2159–2160.

4 O'Brien JT, Erkinjuntti T, Reisberg B, Roman G, Sawada T, Pantoni L, Bowler JV, Ballard C, DeCarli C, Gorelick PB, Rockwood K, Burns A, Gauthier S, DeKosky ST: Vascular cognitive impairment. Lancet Neurol 2003;2:89–98.

5 Ingles JL, Boulton DC, Fisk JD, Rockwood K: Preclinical vascular cognitive impairment and Alzheimer disease: neuropsychological test performance 5 years before diagnosis. Stroke 2007;38: 1148–1153.

6 Petersen RC: Mild cognitive impairment: current research and clinical implications. Semin Neurol 2007;27:22–31.

7 Skoog I, Kalaria RN, Breteler MM: Vascular factors and Alzheimer disease. Alzheimer Dis Assoc Disord 1999;13:S106–S114.

8 Breteler MM: Vascular risk factors for Alzheimer's disease: an epidemiologic perspective. Neurobiol Aging 2000;21:153–160.

9 Román GC: Vascular dementia prevention: a risk factor analysis. Cerebrovasc Dis 2005;20(suppl 2): 91–100.

10 Elias MF, Sullivan LM, D'Agostino RB, Elias PK, Beiser A, Au R, Seshadri S, DeCarli C, Wolf PA: Framingham stroke risk profile and lowered cognitive performance. Stroke 2004;35:404–409.

11 Goldstein LB, Adams R, Alberts MJ, Appel LJ, Brass LM, Bushnell CD, Culebras A, Degraba TJ, Gorelick PB, Guyton JR, Hart RG, Howard G, Kelly-Hayes M, Nixon JV, Sacco RL: Primary prevention of ischemic stroke: a guideline from the American Heart Association/American Stroke Association Stroke Council: cosponsored by the Atherosclerotic Peripheral Vascular Disease Interdisciplinary Working Group; Cardiovascular Nursing Council; Clinical Cardiology Council; Nutrition, Physical Activity, and Metabolism Council, and the Quality of Care and Outcomes Research Interdisciplinary Working Group. Stroke 2006;37:1583–1633.

12 Hankey GJ: Potential new risk factors for ischemic stroke: what is their potential? Stroke 2006;37:2181–2188.

13 Baum LW: Sex, hormones, and Alzheimer's disease. J Gerontol A Biol Sci Med Sci 2005;60:736–743.

14 Qiu C, Winblad B, Fratiglioni L: The age-dependent relation of blood pressure to cognitive function and dementia. Lancet Neurol 2005;4:487–499.
15 Biessels GJ, Staekenborg S, Brunner E, Brayne C, Scheltens P: Risk of dementia in diabetes mellitus: a systematic review. Lancet Neurol 2006;5:64–74.
16 Pasquier F, Boulogne A, Leys D, Fontaine P: Diabetes mellitus and dementia. Diabetes Metab 2006;32:403–414.
17 de Groot JC, de Leeuw FE, Oudkerk M, Hofman A, Jolles J, Breteler MM: Cerebral white matter lesions and subjective cognitive dysfunction: the Rotterdam Scan Study. Neurology 2001;56:1539–1545.
18 Grut M, Jorm AF, Fratiglioni L, Forsell Y, Viitanen M, Winblad B: Memory complaints of elderly people in a population survey: variation according to dementia stage and depression. J Am Geriatr Soc 1993;41:1295–1300.
19 Wang PN, Wang SJ, Fuh JL, Teng EL, Liu CY, Lin CH, Shyu HY, Lu SR, Chen CC, Liu HC: Subjective memory complaint in relation to cognitive performance and depression: a longitudinal study of a rural Chinese population. J Am Geriatr Soc 2000; 48:295–299.
20 St John P, Montgomery P: Is subjective memory loss correlated with MMSE scores or dementia? J Geriatr Psychiatry Neurol 2003;16:80–83.
21 Geerlings MI, Jonker C, Bouter LM, Ader HJ, Schmand B: Association between memory complaints and incident Alzheimer's disease in elderly people with normal baseline cognition. Am J Psychiatry 1999;156:531–537.
22 McGlone J, Gupta S, Humphrey D, Oppenheimer S, Mirsen T, Evans DR: Screening for early dementia using memory complaints from patients and relatives. Arch Neurol 1990;47:1189–1193.
23 Carr DB, Gray S, Baty J, Morris JC: The value of informant versus individual's complaints of memory impairment in early dementia. Neurology 2000;55: 1724–1726.
24 Jorm AF: Methods of screening for dementia: a meta-analysis of studies comparing an informant questionnaire with a brief cognitive test. Alzheimer Dis Assoc Disord 1997;11:158–162.
25 Cacchione PZ, Powlishta KK, Grant EA, Buckles VD, Morris JC: Accuracy of collateral source reports in very mild to mild dementia of the Alzheimer type. J Am Geriatr Soc 2003;51:819–823.
26 Holsinger T, Deveau J, Boustani M, Williams JW Jr: Does this patient have dementia? J Am Med Assoc 2007;297: 2391–2404.
27 Mackinnon A, Mulligan R: Combining cognitive testing and informant report to increase accuracy in screening for dementia. Am J Psychiatry 1998; 155:1529–1535.
28 Tierney MC, Herrmann N, Geslani DM, Szalai JP: Contribution of informant and patient ratings to the accuracy of the Mini-Mental State Examination in predicting probable Alzheimer's disease. J Am Geriatr Soc 2003;51:813–818.
29 Leys D, Hénon H, Mackowiak-Cordoliani MA, Pasquier F: Poststroke dementia. Lancet Neurol 2005;4:752–759.
30 Reitz C, Bos MJ, Hofman A, Koudstaal PJ, Breteler MM: Prestroke cognitive performance, incident stroke, and risk of dementia: the Rotterdam Study. Stroke 2008;39:36–41.
31 Barker-Collo S, Feigin V: The impact of neuropsychological deficits on functional stroke outcomes. Neuropsychol Rev 2006;16:53–64.
32 Nagata K, Saito H, Ueno T, Sato M, Nakase T, Maeda T, Satoh Y, Komatsu H, Suzuki M, Kondoh Y: Clinical diagnosis of vascular dementia. J Neurol Sci 2007;257:44–48.
33 Desmond DW: The neuropsychology of vascular cognitive impairment: is there a specific cognitive deficit? J Neurol Sci 2004;226:3–7.
34 Royall DR, Lauterbach EC, Cummings JL, Reeve A, Rummans TA, Kaufer DI, LaFrance WC Jr, Coffey CE: Executive control function: a review of its promise and challenges for clinical research. A report from the Committee on Research of the American Neuropsychiatric Association. J Neuropsychiatry Clin Neurosci 2002;14:377–405.
35 Pasquier F: Early diagnosis of dementia: neuropsychology. J Neurol 1999;246:6–15.
36 Hachinski V, Iadecola C, Petersen RC, Breteler MM, Nyenhuis DL, Black SE, Powers WJ, DeCarli C, Merino JG, Kalaria RN, Vinters HV, Holtzman DM, Rosenberg GA, Wallin A, Dichgans M, Marler JR, Leblanc GG: National Institute of Neurological Disorders and Stroke-Canadian Stroke Network vascular cognitive impairment harmonization standards. Stroke 2006;37:2220–2241.
37 Folstein M, Folstein S, McHugh PJ: Mini-Mental State: a practical method for grading the cognitive state of patients for clinicians. J Psychiatr Res 1975; 12:189–198.
38 Katz S: Assessing self-maintenance: activities of daily living, mobility, and instrumental activities of daily living. J Am Geriatr Soc 1983;31:721–727.
39 Lawton MP, Brody EM: Assessment of older people: self-maintaining and instrumental activities of daily living. Gerontologist 1969;9:179–186.
40 Gelinàs I, Gauthier L, McIntyre M, et al: Development of a functional measure for persons with Alzheimer's disease: the disability assessment for dementia. Am J Occup Ther 1999;53:471–481.

41 Waldemar G, Dubois B, Emre M, Georges J, McKeith IG, Rossor M, Scheltens P, Tariska P, Winblad B, EFNS: Recommendations for the diagnosis and management of Alzheimer's disease and other disorders associated with dementia: EFNS guideline. Eur J Neurol 2007;14:e1–e26.
42 Galasko D, Bennett D, Sano M, Ernesto C, Thomas R, Grundman M, Ferris S: An inventory to assess activities of daily living for clinical trials in Alzheimer's disease. Alzheimer Dis Assoc Disord 1997; 11(suppl 2):S33–S39.
43 Pfeffer RI, Kurosaki TT, Harrah CH Jr, Chance JM, Filos S: Measurement of functional activities in older adults in the community. J Gerontol 1982;37: 323–329.
44 DeJong R, Osterlund OW, Roy GW: Measurement of quality of life changes in patients with Alzheimer's disease. Clin Ther 1989;11:545–554.
45 Chung JA, Cummings JL: Neurobehavioral and neuropsychiatric symptoms in Alzheimer's disease: characteristics and treatment. Neurol Clin 2000;18: 829–846.
46 Apostolova LG, Cummings JL: Neuropsychiatric manifestations in mild cognitive impairment: a systematic review of the literature. Dement Geriatr Cogn Disord 2008;25:115–126.
47 Hargrave R, Geck LC, Reed B, Mungas D: Affective behavioural disturbances in Alzheimer's disease and ischaemic vascular disease. J Neurol Neurosurg Psychiatry 2000;68:41–46.
48 Srikanth S, Nagaraja AV, Ratnavalli E: Neuropsychiatric symptoms in dementia-frequency, relationship to dementia severity and comparison in Alzheimer's disease, vascular dementia and frontotemporal dementia. J Neurol Sci 2005;236:43–48.
49 Fuh J-L, Wang S-J, Cummings JL: Neuropsychiatric profiles in patients with Alzheimer's disease and vascular dementia. J Neurol Neurosurg Psychiatry 2005;76:1337–1341.
50 Cummings JL, Mega M, Gray K, Rosenberg-Thompson S, Carusi DA, Gornbein J: The Neuropsychiatric Inventory: comprehensive assessment of psychopathology in dementia. Neurology 1994;44:2308–2314.
51 Reisberg B, Borenstein J, Salob SP, Ferris SH, Franssen E, Georgotas A: Behavioral symptoms in Alzheimer's disease: phenomenology and treatment. J Clin Psychiatry 1987;48(suppl 9):9–15.
52 Allen NH, Gordon S, Hope T, Burns A: Manchester and Oxford Universities Scale for the Psychopathological Assessment of Dementia (MOUSEPAD). Br J Psychiatry 1996;169:293–307.
53 Hachinski VC, Iliff LD, Zilhka E, Du Boulay GH, McAllister VL, Marshall J, Russell RW, Symon L: Cerebral blood flow in dementia. Arch Neurol 1975; 32:632–637.
54 Staekenborg SS, van der Flier WM, van Straaten EC, Lane R, Barkhof F, Scheltens P: Neurological signs in relation to type of cerebrovascular disease in vascular dementia. Stroke 2008;39:317–322.
55 Knopman DS, DeKosky ST, Cummings JL, Chui H, Corey-Bloom J, Relkin N, Small GW, Miller B, Stevens JC: Practice parameter: diagnosis of dementia (an evidence-based review). Report of the Quality Standards Subcommittee of the American Academy of Neurology. Neurology 2001;56:1143–1153.
56 Hejl A, Høgh P, Waldemar G: Potentially reversible conditions in 1000 consecutive memory clinic patients. J Neurol Neurosurg Psychiatry 2002;73: 390–394.
57 Clarfield AM: The decreasing prevalence of reversible dementias: an updated meta-analysis. Arch Intern Med 2003;163:2219–2229.
58 Roman GC, Tatemichi TK, Erkinjuntti T, et al: Vascular dementia: diagnostic criteria for research studies. Report of the NINDS-AIREN International Workshop. Neurology 1993;43:250–260.
59 Guermazi A, Miaux Y, Rovira-Cañellas A, Suhy J, Pauls J, Lopez R, Posner H: Neuroradiological findings in vascular dementia. Neuroradiology 2007;49: 1–22.
60 Boustani M, Peterson B, Hanson L, Harris R, Lohr KN: Screening for dementia in primary care: a summary of the evidence for the US preventive services task force. Ann Neurol 2003;138:927–937.

Leonardo Pantoni, MD, PhD
Department of Neurological and Psychiatric Sciences
University of Florence, Viale Morgagni 85
IT–50134 Florence (Italy)
Tel. +39 055 794 7995, Fax +39 055 429 8461, E-Mail pantoni@unifi.it

Giannakopoulos P, Hof PR (eds): Dementia in Clinical Practice.
Front Neurol Neurosci. Basel, Karger, 2009, vol 24, pp 79–85

The Concept of Vascular Cognitive Impairment

Timo Erkinjuntti[a] · Serge Gauthier[b]

[a]Memory Research Unit, Department of Neurology, Helsinki University Central Hospital, Helsinki, Finland;
[b]McGill Center for Studies in Aging, McGill University, Montréal, Que., Canada

Abstract

Vascular cognitive impairment (VCI) is the modern term related to vascular burden of the brain, reflecting all encompassing effects of cerebrovascular disease (CVD) on cognition. VCI include all levels of cognitive decline from mild deficits in one or more cognitive domains to a broad dementia-like syndrome. VCI incorporates the complex interactions between vascular risk factors, CVD etiologies and cellular changes within the brain and cognition. Vascular risk factors towards VCI include, e.g. arterial hypertension, high cholesterol, and diabetes. VCI includes the common poststroke dementia and vascular dementia (VaD). The main subtypes of VaD include the cortical VaD or multi-infarct dementia also referred as poststroke VaD and subcortical ischemic vascular disease and dementia or small vessel dementia. Traditional vascular risk factors and stroke are also independent factors for the clinical presentation of Alzheimer's disease. In addition to these vascular factors, CVD/strokes, infarcts and white matter lesions may trigger and modify progression of Alzheimer's disease. Whilst CVD is preventable and treatable, it clearly is a major factor in the prevalence of cognitive impairment in the elderly worldwide.

Background

Vascular Dementia Concept

During the 1980s and the early 1990s, almost all cerebrovascular injury leading to dementia was ascribed to large cortical and subcortical infarcts, so-called multi infarct dementia (MID) [1]. The concept of vascular dementia (VaD) was introduced to further refine the description of dementias caused by infarcts of varying sizes including the smaller lacunar infarcts and microinfarcts [2]. VaD appropriately defined a group of heterogeneous syndromes of vascular origin of which cortical disease and subcortical vascular disease were considered as important subtypes [3]. Although this was an important step forward, it was not adequate to fully describe the vascular causes of early cognitive impairments.

Concept of Dementia Syndrome
The recognition of Alzheimer's disease (AD) as the commonest cause of dementia led to the development of operational criteria for the diagnosis of dementia in general. The criteria included early and prominent memory loss, progressive cognitive impairment, evidence of irreversibility and presence of cognitive impairment sufficient to affect normal activities of daily living. The characteristic episodic memory impairment apparent in AD is attributed to atrophy of the medial temporal lobe. In contrast, cerebrovascular disease (CVD) lesions do not necessarily have the same regional predilection. The emphasis of the current dementia criteria limited to episodic memory underestimates the vascular burden on cognition. The conventional dementia syndrome concept recognizes the vascular burden of the brain too late, when often opportunities to prevent and treat are lost. Accordingly, it has been suggested that the 'Alzheimerized' dementia concept should be abandoned in the setting of CVD, and indeed this was one of the motives behind development of the broader category of vascular cognitive impairment (VCI) [4, 5].

Modern Concept of Vascular Burden of the Brain: Vascular Cognitive Impairment

VCI Cognitive Syndrome
The cognitive syndrome of VCI encompasses all levels of cognitive decline, from the earliest deficits to a severe and broad dementia-like cognitive syndrome [4, 6]. VCI cases that do not meet the criteria for dementia can also be labeled as VCI with no dementia or vascular cognitive impairment no dementia (vascular CIND). These patients have also been labeled as vascular mild cognitive impairment in a similar way to that of amnestic mild cognitive impairment for AD.

Vascular Cognitive Impairment Pathophysiology
VCI refers to all etiologies of CVD including vascular risks which can result in brain damage leading to cognitive impairment. VCI may include cases with cognitive impairment related to hypertension, diabetes or atherosclerosis, transient ischemic attacks, cortico-subcortical infarcts, silent infarcts, strategic infarcts, small vessel disease with white matter lesions (WMLs) and lacunae, as well as AD pathology with coexisting CVD. VCI can also encompass those patients who survive intracerebral and other intracranial hemorrhages but are left with residual cognitive impairment.

The concept and definition of VCI or vascular CIND are still evolving, but it seems clear that the diagnosis should not be confined to a single etiology comparable to the traditional 'pure AD' concept. The two main factors to be defined in VCI are the severity of cognitive impairment, and the pattern of affected cognitive domains.

Vascular Cognitive Impairment – Size of the Problem

Estimates of the population distribution of VCI and its outcomes are influenced by the variety of definitions used. For example, if AD with CVD or the previously defined VaD with AD pathology is included, then VCI would most certainly be the most common cause of chronic progressive cognitive impairment in elderly people [7]. In the Canadian Study on Health and Aging, the prevalence of VCI has been estimated at 5% in people over age 65 years. These included patients with CIND. The prevalence of vascular CIND, however, was 2.4%, that of AD with CVD was 0.9% and of VaD alone was 1.5%. By comparison, the prevalence of AD without a vascular component, at all ages up to age 85 years, was 5.1% [7].

Risk Factors of Vascular Cognitive Impairment and Dementia

Risk factors associated with VCI include risks for stroke and ischemic WMLs. Clinically symptomatic infarcts, clinically silent infarcts, and WMLs relate to higher dementia risk [8, 9]. Similarly to AD, the risks for VCI may be considered under demographic (e.g. age, education), vascular (e.g. arterial hypertension, atrial fibrillation, myocardial infarction, coronary heart disease, diabetes, generalized atherosclerosis, lipid abnormalities, smoking), genetic (e.g. family history and specific genetic features), and ischemic lesion related variables (e.g. type of CVD, site and size of stroke) [10, 11]. Hypoxic ischemic events (cardiac arrhythmias, congestive heart failure, myocardial infarction, seizures, pneumonia) giving rise to global cerebrovascular insufficiency are important risk factors for incident dementia in patients with stroke [12].

Furthermore the traditional vascular risk factors and stroke are also independent factors for the clinical presentation of mild cognitive impairment and AD [13]. The important independent mid-life risk factors of clinical AD include arterial hypertension, high cholesterol, diabetes, obesity, and reduced physical activity among others [13, 14].

White Matter Lesion Burden

WMLs, frequently detected on neuroimaging, are associated with cognitive, mood, motor, and urinary disorders, all known for contributing towards disability in the elderly [15]. In particular, confluent and extensive WMLs relate to cognitive decline and faster progression of disability. WMLs are seen as the surrogate of small vessel disease and they relate to the subcortical ischemic vascular disease and dementia (SIVD) syndrome [16].

Post-Stroke Cognitive Impairment

Post-stroke cognitive impairment is frequent, as demonstrated in the Helsinki Stroke Ageing Study [17]. Cognitive impairment 3 months after ischemic stroke was present in one domain in 62% and in two domains in 35% of the patients aged 55–85 years. The cognitive domains affected included short-term memory (31%), long-term memory (23%), constructive and visuospatial functions (37%), executive functions (25%) and aphasia (14%) [17].

Post-Stroke Dementia

The frequency of post-stroke dementia vary from 12 to 32% within 3 months to 1 year after stroke [18]. In the Helsinki study, the frequency was 25% 3 months after incident stroke, and the frequency increased with increasing age; 19% among those aged 55–64 years, and 32% in those aged 75–85 years [17].

Determinants of post-stroke dementia include high age, low education, pre-stroke dependency and cognitive impairment [18]. Risk factors of incident post-stroke dementia include epileptic seizures, sepsis, cardiac arrhythmias and congestive heart failure [12, 18]. Brain lesion correlates of post-stroke dementia include a combination of infarct features (volume, site), presence of WMLs (extent, location), as well as brain atrophy [18, 19]. Important critical locations include dominant hemisphere and lesions affecting the prefrontal-subcortical circuit.

Vascular Dementia

VaD, defined as the subset of VCI patients who fulfill the traditional Alzheimer type dementia criteria, is considered the second most common cause of dementia. Using population-based identification of persons aged 65 years and older, the European collaborative study reported that the age-standardized prevalence of dementia was 6.4% (all causes), 4.4% for AD and 1.6% for VaD [20]. In this study 15.8% of all the cases had VaD and 53.7% AD.

VaD as well as VCI encompass many clinical features, which themselves reflect a variety of vascular mechanisms and changes in the brain, with different causes and neurological outcomes. The pathophysiology is attributed to interactions between vascular etiologies (CVD and vascular risk factors), changes in the brain (infarcts, WMLs, atrophy), and host factors (age, education).

The main subtypes of VaD included in current classifications are cortical VaD or MID also referred as poststroke VaD, and SIVD or small vessel dementia and strategic infarct dementia. Hypoperfusion dementia resulting from global cerebrovascular insufficiency is also included. Further, subtypes include strategic infarct dementia, hemorrhagic dementia, hereditary VaD (e.g. CADASIL), and AD with CVD. Most widely used clinical diagnostic criteria for general VaD are the NINDS-AIREN criteria [2]. Research criteria for the SIVD have also been proposed [21].

Small Vessel Disease – Subcortical Ischemic Vascular Disease and Dementia

SIVD incorporates two entities 'the lacunar state' and 'Binswanger's disease' [3]. SIVD is attributed to small vessel disease and is characterized by lacunar infarcts, focal and diffuse ischemic WMLs, and incomplete ischemic injury. Subcortical cognitive syndrome is the cardinal clinical manifestation in SIVD with preferential damage to the prefrontal subcortical circuits [16, 21, 22]. Neuroimaging studies in patients with SIVD reveal multiple lacunes and extensive WMLs, supporting the importance of imaging in the diagnostic criteria [21]. The early cognitive syndrome of SIVD is characterized by a dysexecutive syndrome with slowed information processing, usually mild memory deficit and behavioral symptoms. The dysexecutive syndrome in SIVD includes impairment in goal formulation, initiation, planning, organizing, sequencing, executing, set-shifting and set-maintenance, as well as in abstraction [16, 23]. The memory deficit in SIVD is usually milder than in AD, and is characterized by impaired recall, relative intact recognition, less severe forgetting and better benefit from cues. Behavioral and psychological symptoms in SIVD include depression, personality change, emotional lability and incontinence, as well as inertia, emotional bluntness and psychomotor retardation. Earlier phases of SIVD may include episodes of mild upper motor neuron signs (drift, reflex asymmetry, incoordination), gait disorder (apraxic-ataxic or small-stepped), imbalance and falls, urinary frequency and incontinence, dysarthria, dysphagia as well as extrapyramidal signs such as hypokinesia and rigidity [3]. However, these focal neurological signs are often subtle.

Cortical Vascular Dementia

Cortical VaD (MID, poststroke VaD) has been traditionally characterized by a relatively abrupt onset (days to weeks), a stepwise deterioration (some recovery after worsening), and a fluctuating course (e.g. difference between days) of cognitive functions [1, 2, 24, 25]. Cortical VaD relates predominantly to large vessel disease and cardiac embolic events. It is characterized by predominantly cortical and cortico-subcortical arterial territorial and distal field (watershed) infarcts. The early cognitive syndrome of cortical VaD includes some memory impairment, which may be mild, and some heteromodal cortical symptom(s) such as aphasia, apraxia, agnosia and visuospatial or constructional difficulty. In addition, most patients have some degree of dysexecutive syndrome. Due to the multiple cortico-subcortical infarcts, patients with cortical VaD often have additional neurological deficits such as visual field deficits, lower facial weakness, lateralized sensorimotor changes and gait impairment [25].

Alzheimer's Disease with Cerebrovascular Disease

AD and CVD coexist in a large proportion of patients. Further, CVD also plays an important role in determining the presence and severity of clinical symptoms of AD [26]. AD with CVD can present clinically either as AD with evidence of vascular lesions upon brain imaging or with clinical features of both AD and VaD [27]. In a Canadian study, typical AD presentations with one or more features pointing to 'vascular aspects' derived from the Hachinski Ischemic Scale [28], were used successfully to diagnose AD plus CVD in combination with neuroimaging of ischemic lesions [7]. Vascular risk factors, and focal neurological signs were present more often in AD with CVD than in 'pure' AD. Other clinical clues for a diagnosis of AD with CVD were gained from analyses of disease course characteristics and presentations of patchy cognitive deficits, early onset of seizures and gait disorder. A better solution to recognizing patients with AD plus CVD would be to discover reliable biological markers of clinical AD. Other potential markers include early prominent episodic memory impairment, early and significant medial temporal lobe atrophy on MRI, bilateral parietal hypoperfusion on single photon emission computed tomography and low concentrations of cerebrospinal fluid Aβ peptides with high tau protein.

Conclusions

VCI is a modification of the terminology related to vascular burden of the brain, reflecting the all encompassing effects of CVD on cognition. VCI incorporates the complex interactions between vascular etiologies, risk factors and cellular changes within the brain and cognition. VCI refers to all etiologies of CVD including vascular risks which can result in brain damage leading to cognitive impairment. VCI may include cases with cognitive impairment related to hypertension, diabetes or atherosclerosis, transient ischemic attacks, multiple corticosubcortical infarcts, silent infarcts, strategic infarcts, small vessel disease with WMLs and lacunae, as well as AD pathology with coexisting CVD.

The impairment encompasses all levels of cognitive decline, from the earliest deficits to a severe and broad dementia like cognitive syndrome. The concept and definition of VCI are still evolving, but the diagnosis should not be confined to a single etiology comparable to the traditional 'pure AD' concept. The two main factors to be defined in VCI are the severity of cognitive impairment, and the pattern of affected cognitive domains. Early recognition of VCI will open new prospects for prevention and treatment of the vascular burden of the brain, which is currently done primarily by controlling vascular risk factors.

References

1 Erkinjuntti T, Hachinski VC: Rethinking vascular dementia. Cerebrovasc Dis 1993;3:3–23.

2 Roman GC, Tatemichi TK, Erkinjuntti T, et al: Vascular dementia: diagnostic criteria for research studies. Report of the NINDS-AIREN International Work Group. Neurology 1993;43:250–260.

3 Roman GC, Erkinjuntti T, Wallin A, Pantoni L, Chui HC: Subcortical ischaemic vascular dementia. Lancet Neurol 2002;1:426–436.

4 O'Brien JT, Erkinjuntti T, Reisberg B, et al: Vascular cognitive impairment. Lancet Neurol 2003;2:89–98.

5 Roman GC, Sachdev P, Royall DR, et al: Vascular cognitive disorder: a new diagnostic category updating vascular cognitive impairment and vascular dementia. J Neurol Sci 2004;226:81–87.

6 Bowler JV, Steenhuis R, Hachinski V: Conceptual background of vascular cognitive impairment. Alzheimer Dis Assoc Disord 1999;13:S30–S37.

7 Rockwood K, Wenzel C, Hachinski V, Hogan DB, MacKnight C, McDowell I: Prevalence and outcomes of vascular cognitive impairment. Neurology 2000;54:447–451.

8 Vermeer SE, Prins ND, den Heijer T, Hofman A, Kloudstaal PJ, Breteler MM: Silent brain infarcts and the risk of dementia and cognitive decline. N Engl J Med 2003;348:1215–1222.

9 Prins ND, van Dijk EJ, den Heijer T, et al: Cerebral white matter lesions and the risk of dementia. Arch Neurol 2004;61:1503–1504.

10 Gorelick PB: Status of risk factors for dementia associated with stroke. Stroke 1997;28:459–463.

11 Skoog I: Status of risk factors for vascular dementia. Neuroepidemiology 1998;17:2–9.

12 Moroney JT, Bagiella E, Desmond DW, Paik MC, Stern Y, Tatemichi TK: Risk factors for incident dementia after stroke. Role of hypoxic and ischemic disorders. Stroke 1996;27:1283–1289.

13 Skoog I, Kalaria RN, Breteler MMB: Vascular factors and Alzheimer's disease. Alzheimer Dis Assoc Disord 1999;13:S106–S114.

14 Kivpelto M, Ngandu T, Laatikainen T, Winblad B, Soininen H, Tuomilehto J: Risk score for the prediction of dementia risk in 20 years among middle aged people: a longitudinal, population-based study. Lancet Neurol 2006;5:735–741.

15 Inzitari D, Simoni M, Paracucci G, et al: Risk of rapid global functional decline in elderly patients with severe cerebral age-related white matter changes: the LADIS Study. Arch Intern Med 2007;167:81–88.

16 Jokinen H, Kalska H, Mäntylä R, et al: Cognitive profile of subcortical vascular disease. J Neurol Neurosurg Psychiatry 2006;77:28–33.

17 Pohjasvaara T, Erkinjuntti T, Vataja R, Kaste M: Dementia three months after stroke. Baseline frequency and effect of different definitions of dementia in the Helsinki Stroke Aging Memory Study (SAM) cohort. Stroke 1997;28:785–792.

18 Leys D, Henon H, Mackowiak-Cordoliani M-A, Pasquier F: Poststroke dementia. Lancet Neurol 2005;4:752–759.

19 Pohjasvaara T, Mäntylä R, Salonen O, et al: How complex interactions of ischemic brain infarcts, white matter lesions and atrophy relate to poststroke dementia. Arch Neurol 2000;57:1295–1300.

20 Lobo A, Launer LJ, Fratiglioni L, et al: Prevalence of dementia and major subtypes in Europe: a collaborative study of population-based cohorts. Neurology 2000;54:S4–S9.

21 Erkinjuntti T, Inzitari D, Pantoni L, et al: Research criteria for subcortical vascular dementia in clinical trials. J Neural Transm 2000;59:23–30.

22 Cummings JL: Fronto-subcortical circuits and human behavior. Arch Neurol 1993;50:873–880.

23 Cummings JL: Vascular subcortical dementias: clinical aspects. Dementia 1994;5:177–180.

24 Chui HC, Victoroff JI, Margolin D, Jagust W, Shankle R, Katzman R: Criteria for the diagnosis of ischemic vascular dementia proposed by the State of California Alzheimer's Disease Diagnostic and Treatment Centers. Neurology 1992;42:473–480.

25 Erkinjuntti T: Types of multi-infarct dementia. Acta Neurol Scand 1987;75:391–399.

26 Snowdon DA, Greiner LH, Mortimer JA, Riley KP, Greiner PA, Markesbery WR: Brain infarction and the clinical expression of Alzheimer disease. The Nun Study. J Am Med Assoc 1997;277:813–817.

27 Rockwood K, Howard K, MacKnight C, Darvesh S: Spectrum of disease in vascular cognitive impairment. Neuroepidemiology 1999;18:248–254.

28 Hachinski VC, Iliff LD, Zilhka E, et al: Cerebral blood flow in dementia. Arch Neurol 1975;32:632–637.

Prof. Timo Erkinjuntti
Memory Research Unit, Department of Neurology
Helsinki University Central Hospital
PO Box 300, FI–00029 Helsinki (Finland)
Tel. +358 40 5000 827, Fax +358 94 7172 352, E-Mail Timo.Erkinjuntti@hus.fi

Giannakopoulos P, Hof PR (eds): Dementia in Clinical Practice.
Front Neurol Neurosci. Basel, Karger, 2009, vol 24, pp 86–94

Defining the Neuropathological Background of Vascular and Mixed Dementia and Comparison with Magnetic Resonance Imaging Findings

Gabriel Gold

Department of Geriatrics and Rehabilitation, Geneva University School of Medicine and Geneva University Hospitals, Thônex, Geneva, Switzerland

Abstract

The concept of vascular dementia (VaD) has greatly evolved in the past decades. Advances in neuroimaging techniques have led to a better identification of cases with small vessel disease and chronic ischemic changes. Autopsy data from population-based studies have revealed the frequent occurrence of both vascular and degenerative lesions in aged brains. However, the clinical significance of vascular pathology has been difficult to establish. This chapter will review data from clinicoradiological and clinicopathological studies that have attempted to define the cognitive impact of macroscopic and microscopic ischemic pathology in pure VaD and in cases with associated degenerative pathology. Magnetic resonance imaging studies have focused on lacunes and white matter lesions, whereas autopsy series have provide important insights into the clinical correlates of macroinfarcts, lacunes, diffuse and periventricular demyelination, microinfarcts and focal and diffuse gliosis. Results from these studies have led to a better understanding of the influence of lesion type, location and severity on cognitive function. Vascular scores have been proposed that can be combined with well-established classifications of Alzheimer's disease (AD) pathology to distinguish mixed dementias from pure AD and pure VaD.

The consequences of apoplexy on intellectual function were described in ancient times but the first reports clearly linking cerebral softening, arteriosclerosis and vascular occlusion date back to the early and mid-19th century. In the late 19th century, Binswanger described three major forms of dementia related to vascular pathology: (1) encephalitis subcorticalis chronica progressiva associated with severe white matter atrophy and ventricular enlargement without any evidence of focal disease, (2) arteriosclerotic brain degeneration which presented with widespread large artery arteriosclerosis and cortical and white matter discoloration and (3) dementia postapoplexiam which was characterized by acute onset and focal deficits. Alzheimer described glial proliferation and scarring in encephalitis chronica progressiva and senile cortical atrophy associated with wedge-shaped cortical infarcts and softened convolutions with many punctuate indentations [1]. These descriptions did not include precise clinicopathological correlations, provided no information on the relationship between clinical findings and lesion type, severity and location, and thus were unable to fully validate the contribution of the above lesions to the development of intellectual dysfunction of vascular origin.

During the 20th century, emphasis was first put on arteriosclerosis of cerebral blood vessels without a clear description of the exact lesion responsible for cognitive changes, but soon stroke was felt to be the major cause of vascular dementia (VaD). Later, the concept evolved to include multiple physiopathological mechanisms related to deficiencies in blood supply including large vessel disease, small vessel pathology, consequences of cerebral hypoperfusion and hemorrhage. Complicating matters further, the pathological examination of older brains in large community samples revealed a high frequency of vascular lesions even in the absence of dementia. These include macroinfarcts, lacunes, demyelination, gliosis and cortical microinfarcts (fig. 1). Over three quarters of autopsies performed in participants of the Medical Research Council Cognitive Function and Ageing Study (mean age at death of 85 years for men and 86 years for women) showed cerebrovascular pathology, and 95% of postmortem magnetic resonance imaging (MRI) scans exhibited white matter lesions (WML) [2, 3]. In this study, cerebral vascular lesions were common in both demented and nondemented individuals, although multiple lesions were more frequent in the former group.

The development of universally recognized clinical and neuropathological criteria for VaD has been greatly hampered by the lack of precise information linking specific lesions to intellectual dysfunction. This chapter will attempt to answer several key questions: (1) Among the numerous vascular lesions encountered in older brains, which ones are important from a cognitive point of view? (2) Which characteristics of these lesions are the best correlates of intellectual function (location, size or type)? (3) Can neuroimaging and neuropathology help define the broad spectrum of mixed dementia (MD) and its extremes (pure VaD and pure Alzheimer's disease, AD)?

Brain Macroinfarcts and Post-Stroke Dementia

VaD has long been thought to result from cerebral infarction based on a large body of epidemiological data. From a neuropathological point of view, this concept was established in part by the landmark studies of Tomlinson who demonstrated the importance of infarct size. In his experience, cerebral softening of 50 ml or more occurred in one third of demented individuals but only rarely in nondemented people. He also showed that dementia was always present when 100 ml or more of brain tissue were damaged due to stroke [4, 5].

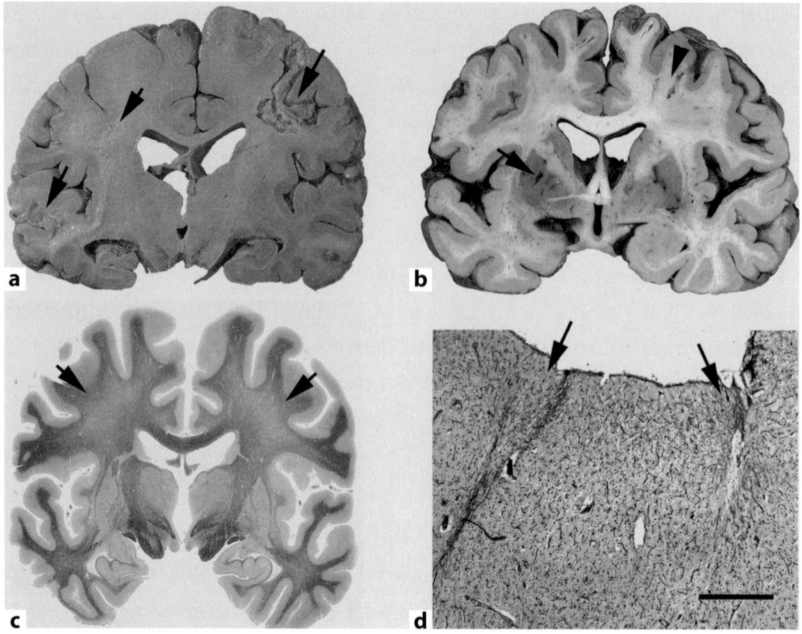

Fig. 1. **a** Multiple brain infarcts. **b** Lacune in the putamen (arrow) and in the frontal white matter (arrowhead). **c** Deep white matter demyelination. **d** Cortical microinfarct scars (Globus silver impregnation). Scale bar (for **d**) 700 µm.

The term multi-infarct dementia was later introduced by Hachinski to describe the intellectual consequences of multiple strokes of thromboembolic origin and led to the development of the ischemic score that is still used in some studies today [6]. In this concept, the number and location of strokes was felt to be more important than the actual volume of affected tissue.

Although VaD can be described as a consequence of an acute ischemic event, it is important to note that individuals with stroke are at much higher risk of developing intellectual impairment during the following years [7]. This raises an important issue: is the delayed onset of dementia due to repeat stroke, concomitant neurodegenerative disease or an associated chronic ischemic process?

Microscopic Infarcts

Several authors have suggested that microscopic ischemic pathology may be more important than large infarcts in the development of dementia. In one series of 130 older individuals, microinfarcts were more common in severely demented and cognitively impaired cases than in aged controls without cognitive impairment as opposed to large infarcts which were more common in the latter group [8]. In another study of elderly autopsied cases with mild to moderate AD and controls, the presence of microvascular cerebral pathology was correlated with dementia [9]. Unfortunately, the cognitive impact of microscopic infarcts has been difficult to define since such lesions are diffusely developed within the brain and may be inadequately assessed when a standard neuropathological examination is performed. Their evaluation requires systematic bilateral examination of cortical regions known to be highly involved in dementia such as the hippocampus and neocortical association areas. Furthermore, concomitant vascular or degenerative lesions may mask the effect of microscopic infarcts.

This issue has been addressed in an autopsy series of 45 elderly individuals with vascular pathology confined to microvascular infarcts, gliosis and demyelination that excluded cases with significant neurodegenerative pathology. Cortical microinfarcts proved to be the most powerful correlate of cognitive status in both univariate and multivariate analyses with a clear association between the severity of the microinfarct score and the level of global cognitive function [10]. Focal cortical and white matter gliosis were not related to the clinical findings.

Lacunes

Lacunes are commonly encountered in the brains of older people and may represent the most frequent type of cerebrovascular lesion [11]. The clinical expression of lacunes has been the source of conflicting reports. In a large cross-sectional MRI study of AD and subcortical ischemic VaD, volume of lacunes was not a significant correlate of cognitive measures [12] However, in a follow-up 3-year longitudinal study lacunar volume did not predict global cognition but did seem to modulate the clinical consequences of decreased hippocampal volume [13]. Interestingly, lacunes appeared to have a small effect on executive function but not on memory [14]. In a relatively rare familial form of VaD, cerebral autosomal dominant arteriopathy with subcortical infarcts and leukoencephalopathy, lacunes were the main MRI correlate of cognitive dysfunction [15].

In a large neuropathological study, lacunes were found in one quarter of cognitively intact elderly [16]. In contrast, the nun study clearly demonstrated the important influence of lacunes on the occurrence of dementia when AD pathology is also present [17]. From a neuropathological point of view, the assessment of lacunes raises issues similar to those discussed above for microinfarcts, bilateral evaluation of regions known to be important for cognition is necessary but standard neuropathological procedures usually do not include such an approach [18]. An autopsy series of older individuals that applied such a method and included cases with lacunes and demyelination but excluded macroinfarcts and significant neurofibrillary tangle formation (Braak stage higher than II excluded), illustrated the importance of location as well as lesion type in determining the cognitive consequences of vascular pathology. Lacunes in frontal, parietal and temporal deep white matter were unrelated to cognitive status as opposed to lacunes in the thalamus and basal ganglia that exhibited a clear relationship between severity of lacunar pathology and global cognitive function. Interestingly, multivariate analysis showed that microinfarcts remained stronger predictors of cognitive status than both thalamic and basal ganglia lacunes [19].

Periventricular and Diffuse Demyelination

The ever-increasing use of modern neuroimaging methods has led to the increased recognition of WML. Although they are particularly common in the elderly, their clinical significance is unclear. Their presence has been associated with cognitive impairment and depression, but MRI-based studies have shown that they also occur in individuals with normal cognitive function and that age is the strongest predictor of the presence and severity of cerebral WML [20]. They are anatomically divided into periventricular and deep subcortical WML, and some studies have suggested that their consequences on cerebral cognitive and affective function may depend on their location. In the Rotterdam Scan Study of 1,077 community-dwelling elderly, periventricular WML were related to global cognitive function, but subcortical WML were not [21]. In a study of individuals with AD, periventricular WML were associated with impaired executive function and subcortical WML with depressed mood [22]. However, recent data have shown that periventricular and deep white matter hyperintensities are highly correlated with each other, which may explain some of the difficulties encountered when trying to identify their differential effect on cognition [23]. There also appears to be a threshold effect that modulates the pattern of neuropsychological impairment. Cases with mild WML have lower scores on tests of episodic memory, whereas patients with severe WML have lower scores on tests of working memory [24].

WML and lacunes often coexist, and their independent contribution to cognitive function can be difficult to establish. In a study of 46 patients with newly discovered lacunar stroke, the presence of leukoaraiosis was associated with worse cognitive function [25]. Other MRI studies using multivariate analyses have reported that WML remain weak independent predictors of cognitive status and longitudinal decline but not lacunar volume [12, 13]. Interestingly, this contrasts with neuropathological studies discussed below with opposite results. In this regard, it is important to note that WML identified by neuroimaging correspond to variable combinations of myelin and axonal loss, scattered microinfarcts, astrogliosis and dilatation of periventricular spaces and that neuropathology remains the most specific approach for the identification of demyelination [26, 27].

Two autopsy series that excluded cases with macroinfarcts or significant neurofibrillary tangle pathology reported that both periventricular and deep subcortical demyelination were related to cognition [10, 19]. In the first study, periventricular WML were more closely correlated to clinical findings, but in the second study both types of WML contributed equally to global cognitive dysfunction. In multivariate analyses, demyelination was the weakest independent correlate of global cognitive function and was no longer a significant factor after controlling for the presence of lacunes.

Interaction with Alzheimer's Disease Lesions: Pure and Mixed Dementias

MD occurs when Alzheimer pathology and cerebral vascular lesions both lead to the presence of cognitive impairment. As AD and VaD are the most common causes of dementia in the elderly, it is not surprising that they often coexist. However, the interaction between degenerative and vascular pathology and their relative contribution to the occurrence of dementia has been difficult to define. This is complicated by the fact that MD represents a large spectrum of disease between cases with marked AD pathology and few vascular lesions at one extreme and cases with severe vascular pathology and minimal AD changes at the other. In advanced stages of AD, the neurodegenerative pathology appears to overwhelm the cognitive effect of associated vascular lesions [28]. On the other hand, the study of borderline cases (Braak III neurofibrillary tangle stage) at high risk for dementia confirmed the cognitive impact of cortical microinfarcts and periventricular demyelination [29].

From a structural radiological perspective, medial temporal atrophy is generally considered to be the best surrogate marker of degenerative pathology in AD. In cases with both small vessel disease and medial temporal atrophy, the latter appears to be the stronger predictor of the presence of dementia [12, 30, 31]. A recent multivariate analysis of MRI findings in MD has reported that both medial temporal atrophy and large vessel disease contribute to global cognitive impairment, whereas the cognitive impact of white matter hyperintensities was restricted to certain tests of executive function (symbol digit modalities and digit cancellation) and that of multiple lacunar infarcts and thalamic lesions to worse verbal fluency [32].

From a neuropathological point of view, lacunes and small vessel disease are particularly important determinants of cognitive impairment in people with AD lesions [33]. In a large autopsy series of 148 aged individuals, the odds for dementia were increased fourfold in cases with AD pathology in the presence of cortical infarcts; a similar fourfold increase also occurred in the presence of subcortical infarcts [34]. More than half of the subjects with macroscopic infarcts also had microscopic infarcts; the latter were not separately related to dementia in this series. It is likely that the presence of concomitant macroscopic pathology may have masked the cognitive consequences of microscopic lesions. This is supported by another evaluation of 156 autopsied elderly subjects with varying degrees of AD, lacunar and microvascular pathology but without macrovascular infarcts [35]. In this study, cortical microinfarcts and thalamic and basal ganglia lacunes were all significant correlates of cognitive function. Again, frontal, temporal and parietal white matter lacunes,

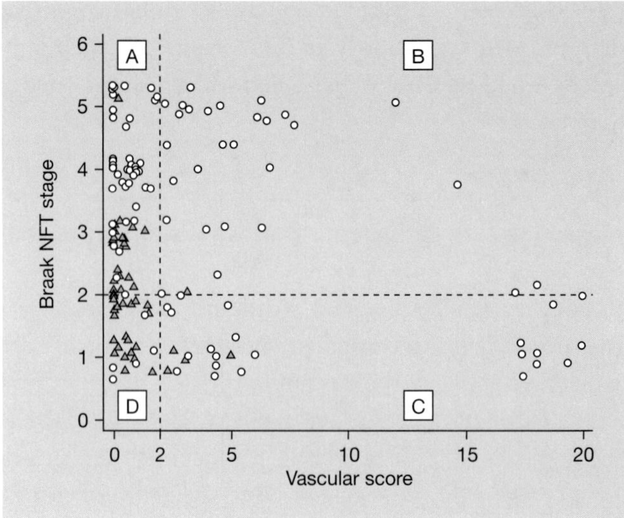

Fig. 2. Scatterplot of demented (open circles) and nondemented (grey triangles) cases according to Braak NFT stage and vascular score. The thresholds determined by sensitivity analysis (dotted lines) delineate four sectors. Demented cases are consistent with pure AD in sector A, pure VaD in sector C, and MD in sector B; most cases in sector D are not demented. In order to avoid superimposition of multiple cases, a 10% random noise was applied to all points. Reprinted with permission from Gold et al. [35].

periventricular and diffuse white matter demyelination and focal and diffuse cortical gliosis were not associated with cognition in multivariate analyses. The authors developed thresholds for vascular and degenerative pathology based on neurofibrillary Braak staging on the one hand and microinfarcts and thalamic and basal ganglia on the other that were able to predict the presence of dementia with great accuracy and provided a strong basis for distinguishing pure VaD or AD from mixed cases (fig. 2).

Conclusion

Clinicoradiological and clinicopathological studies have led to a better understanding of the various lesions involved in the development of vascular and mixed dementias. Although large vessel disease leading to strategic or multiple infarcts is a well established form of VaD, it appears that small vessel disease and chronic ischemia are probably the most common underlying pathology in VaD. Microinfarcts seem to be the most powerful correlate of cognitive status in cases without macroscopic infarcts. It is important to note that microinfarcts are not visible in vivo through neuroimaging modalities, which suggests that a number of cases clinically diagnosed as pure AD may in fact represent cases of MD resulting from both neurodegeneration and microscopic ischemic pathology. Data on lacunes illustrate the importance of lesion location in determining the cognitive consequences of cerebral vascular pathology. In fact, AD cases associated with lacunes confined to frontal, parietal and temporal white matter should not be diagnosed as MD; in such situations, the cognitive deterioration should be attributed solely to the degenerative pathology. The cognitive impact of WML remains difficult to define. Neuropathological evaluation is particularly important for the evaluation of such lesions as it has the advantage of a more precise identification of demyelination compared to neuroimaging techniques. Postmortem morphological examination clearly shows that both periventricular and deep subcortical WML may be associated with cognitive changes, but this relationship does not appear to be very robust. Since lacunes and WML often coexist, each may mask the other's effect. In contrast to reports based on neuroimaging series, multivariate analyses of neuropathological data strongly suggest that lacunes are the stronger determinant of cognitive function.

Clinicopathological studies in AD have demonstrated that neurofibrillary tangle staging is a strong correlate of cognitive function in this disease and that amyloid staging does not have any significant additional power to predict clinical findings. It has been possible to build on this information, incorporating results of recent studies outlining the clinical impact of lacunes and microscopic ischemic pathology and propose a simple semiquantitative vascular score that can be used with Braak neurofibrillary tangle staging to develop neuropathological criteria for MD.

References

1 Mast H, Tatemichi TK, Mohr JP: Chronic brain ischemia: the contributions of Otto Binswanger and Alois Alzheimer to the mechanisms of vascular dementia. J Neurol Sci 1995;132:4–10.
2 Neuropathology group of the medical research council cognitive function and ageing study (MRC CFAS): Pathological correlates of late-onset dementia in a multicentre, community-based population in England and Wales. Lancet 2001;357:169–175.
3 Fernando MS, Ince PG: Vascular pathologies and cognition in a population-based cohort of elderly people. J Neurol Sci 2004;226:13–17.
4 Tomlinson BE, Blessed G, Roth M: Observations on the brains of non-demented old people. J Neurol Sci 1968;7:331–356.
5 Tomlinson BE, Blessed G, Roth M: Observations on the brains of demented old people. J Neurol Sci 1970;11:205–242.
6 Hachinski VD, Lassen NA, Marshall J: Multi-infarct dementia. A cause of mental deterioration in the elderly. Lancet 1974;2:207–210.
7 Desmond DW, Moroney JT, Sano M, Stern Y: Incidence of dementia after ischemic stroke: results of a longitudinal study. Stroke 2002;33:2254–2260.
8 Jellinger KA: Understanding the pathology of vascular cognitive impairment. J Neurol Sci 2005;229–230:57–63.
9 Esiri MM, Wilcock GK, Morris JH: Neuropathological assessment of the lesions of significance in vascular dementia. J Neurol Neurosurg Psychiatry 1997;63:749–753.
10 Kövari E, Gold G, Herrmann FR, Canuto A, Hof PR, Michel JP, Bouras C, Giannakopoulos P: Cortical microinfarcts and demyelination significantly affect cognition in brain aging. Stroke 2004; 35:410–414.
11 Jellinger KA: The enigma of vascular cognitive disorder and vascular dementia. Acta Neuropathol 2007;113:349–388.
12 Mungas D, Jagust WJ, Reed BR, Kramer JH, Weiner MW, Schuff N, Norman D, Mack WJ, Willis L, Chui HC: MRI predictors of cognition in subcortical ischemic vascular disease and Alzheimer's disease. Neurology 2001;57:2229–2235.
13 Mungas D, Reed BR, Jagust WJ, DeCarli C, Mack WJ, Kramer JH, Weiner MW, Schuff N, Chui HC: Volumetric MRI predicts rate of cognitive decline related to AD and cerebrovascular disease. Neurology 2002;59:867–873.
14 Mungas D, Harvey D, Reed BR, Jagust WJ, DeCarli C, Beckett L, Mack WJ, Kramer JH, Weiner MW, Schuff N, Chui HC: Longitudinal volumetric MRI change and rate of cognitive decline. Neurology 2005; 65:565–571.
15 Liem MK, van der Grond J, Haan J, van den Boom R, Ferrari MD, Knaap YM, Breuning MH, van Buchem MA, Middelkoop HA, Lesnik Oberstein SA: Lacunar infarcts are the main correlate with cognitive dysfunction in CADASIL. Stroke 2007;38: 923–928.
16 Jellinger KA, Attems J: Incidence of cerebrovascular lesions in Alzheimer's disease: a postmortem study. Acta Neuropathol (Berl) 2003;105:14–17.

17 Snowdon DA, Greiner LH, Mortimer JA, Riley KP, Greiner PA, Markesbery WR: Brain infarction and the clinical expression of Alzheimer disease. The nun study. J Am Med Assoc 1997;277:813–817.
18 Pantoni L, Sarti C, Alafuzoff I, Jellinger K, Munoz DG, Ogata J, Palumbo V: Postmortem examination of vascular lesions in cognitive impairment: a survey among neuropathological services. Stroke 2006; 37:1005–1009.
19 Gold G, Kövari E, Herrmann FR, Canuto A, Hof PR, Michel JP, Bouras C, Giannakopoulos P: Cognitive consequences of thalamic, basal ganglia, and deep white matter lacunes in brain aging and dementia. Stroke 2005;36:1184–1188.
20 Chui HC: Subcortical ischemic vascular dementia. Neurol Clin 2007;25:717–740.
21 Prins ND, van Dijk EJ, den Heijer T, Vermeer SE, Jolles J, Koudstaal PJ, Hofman A, Breteler MM: Cerebral small-vessel disease and decline in information processing speed, executive function and memory. Brain 2005;128:2034–2041.
22 Bracco L, Piccini C, Moretti M, Mascalchi M, Sforza A, Nacmias B, Cellini E, Bagnoli S, Sorbi S: Alzheimer's disease: role of size and location of white matter changes in determining cognitive deficits. Dement Geriatr Cogn Disord 2005;20:358–366.
23 Swartz RH, Stuss DT, Gao F, Black SE: Independent cognitive effects of atrophy and diffuse subcortical and thalamico-cortical cerebrovascular disease in dementia. Stroke 2008;39:822–830.
24 Libon DJ, Price CC, Giovannetti T, Swenson R, Bettcher BM, Heilman KM, Pennisi A: Linking MRI hyperintensities with patterns of neuropsychological impairment: evidence for a threshold effect. Stroke 2008;39:806–813.
25 McMurtray AM, Liao A, Haider J, Licht E, Mendez MF: Cognitive performance after lacunar stroke correlates with leukoaraiosis severity. Cerebrovasc Dis 2007;24:271–276.
26 Jagust WJ, Zheng L, Harvey DJ, Mack WJ, Vinters HV, Weiner MW, Ellis WG, Zarow C, Mungas D, Reed BR, Kramer JH, Schuff N, DeCarli C, Chui HC: Neuropathological basis of magnetic resonance images in aging and dementia. Ann Neurol 2008; 63:72–80.
27 Udaka F, Sawada H, Kameyama M: White matter lesions and dementia: MRI-pathological correlation. Ann N Y Acad Sci 2002;977:411–415.
28 Jellinger KA: Morphologic diagnosis of 'vascular dementia' – a critical update. J Neurol Sci 2008; 270: 1–12.
29 Kövari E, Gold G, Herrmann FR, Canuto A, Hof PR, Bouras C, Giannakopoulos P: Cortical microinfarcts and demyelination affect cognition in cases at high risk for dementia. Neurology 2007;68:927–931.
30 Fein G, Di Sclafani V, Tanabe J, Cardenas V, Weiner MW, Jagust WJ, Reed BR, Norman D, Schuff N, Kusdra L, Greenfield T, Chui H: Hippocampal and cortical atrophy predict dementia in subcortical ischemic vascular disease. Neurology 2000;55:1626–1635.
31 Du AT, Schuff N, Laakso MP, Zhu XP, Jagust WJ, Yaffe K, Kramer JH, Miller BL, Reed BR, Norman D, Chui HC, Weiner MW: Effects of subcortical ischemic vascular dementia and AD on entorhinal cortex and hippocampus. Neurology 2002;58:1635–1641.
32 Bastos-Leite AJ, van der Flier WM, van Straaten EC, Staekenborg SS, Scheltens P, Barkhof F: The contribution of medial temporal lobe atrophy and vascular pathology to cognitive impairment in vascular dementia. Stroke 2007;38:3182–3185.
33 Jellinger KA, Attems J: Neuropathological evaluation of mixed dementia. J Neurol Sci 2007;257: 80–87.
34 Schneider JA, Boyle PA, Arvanitakis Z, Bienias JL, Bennett DA: Subcortical infarcts, Alzheimer's disease pathology, and memory function in older persons. Ann Neurol 2007;62:59–66.
35 Gold G, Giannakopoulos P, Herrmann FR, Bouras C, Kövari E: Identification of Alzheimer and vascular lesion thresholds for mixed dementia. Brain 2007;130:2830–2836.

Prof. Gabriel Gold
Department of Geriatrics and Rehabilitation, Hôpital des Trois-Chênes
3, chemin du Pont-Bochet
CH–1226 Thônex, Geneva (Switzerland)
Tel. +41 22 305 6530, Fax +41 22 305 6528, E-Mail Gabriel.gold@hcuge.ch

Giannakopoulos P, Hof PR (eds): Dementia in Clinical Practice.
Front Neurol Neurosci. Basel, Karger, 2009, vol 24, pp 95–106

Is It Possible to Treat Vascular Dementia?

Dina Zekry

Department of Rehabilitation and Geriatrics, Geneva University Hospitals and University of Geneva, Thônex, Geneva, Switzerland

Abstract

Randomized controlled trials of primary and secondary prevention of vascular dementia demonstrate real effects on the cause or progression of disease (disease-modifying treatment). These strategies lead to a reduction in all cerebrovascular risk factors, in particular hypertension. Such treatment may prevent dementia by reducing stroke and possibly by other mechanisms that remain undetermined, such as those involved in neurodegeneration and cell death. Curative treatment of vascular dementia, particularly given recent studies on cholinesterase inhibitors (rivastigmine, donepezil and galantamine) and memantine, is still ineffective. There is insufficient evidence to support widespread use of these drugs in vascular dementia. Particular considerations should be taken into account in clinical trials. Vascular dementia is a heterogeneous disease with different subtypes and mechanisms. Therefore, well-designed, adequately powered trials accounting for this heterogeneity, with better clinical definitions and an assessment and detection of cognitive and global changes specific to vascular dementia, are needed.

The Three Main Objectives in the Treatment of Vascular Dementia

Prevention

Before Stroke (Primary Prevention)

One of the most promising lines of research involves trials of preventive treatment in individuals with multiple risk factors: smokers, diabetics, atrial fibrillation, cardiac and hypertensive patients. In addition, recent epidemiological studies suggest that primary prevention of dementia in such patients should be applied from midlife. A retrospective cohort study was carried out, involving 8,845 participants from a health maintenance organization undergoing health evaluations between 1964 and 1973, between the ages of 40 and 44. Midlife cardiovascular risk factors included total cholesterol, diabetes, hypertension, and smoking. Diagnoses of dementia were ascertained from medical records between January 1994 and April 2003. The authors identified 721 participants (8.2%) with dementia. Smoking, hypertension, high cholesterol, and diabetes at midlife were each associated with an increase in risk of dementia of between 20 and 40% (fully adjusted Cox proportional hazards model: HR 1.24, 95% confidence interval (CI) 1.04–1.48 for hypertension, HR 1.26, 95% CI 1.08–1.47 for smoking, HR 1.42, 95% CI 1.22–1.66 for high cholesterol, and HR 1.46, 95% CI 1.19–1.79 for diabetes). A composite cardiovascular risk score was created using all four risk factors and was associated with dementia in a dose-dependent fashion. Compared with participants having no risk factors, the risk for dementia increased from 1.27 for having one risk factor to 2.37 for having all four risk factors [1]. In this study, the presence of multiple cardiovascular risk factors at midlife substantially increased risk of late-life dementia in a dose-dependent manner. It thus remains to be shown that interventions targeting these risk factors – giving up smoking; control of diabetes, hyperlipidemia and obesity; carotid endarterectomy for symptomatic patients with 70–99% carotid stenosis; anticoagulants for atrial fibrillation; aspirin for patients at high primary risk and antihypertensives – would allow reduction of the risk of later development of dementia. Only a few studies of intervention exist. In the SHEP study [2], treatment of isolated systolic hypertension in individuals over the age of 60 years led to a 36% reduction in the incidence of stroke. The SYST-EUR trial [3] reported a 42% reduction in the overall incidence rate for stroke using antihypertensive treatment in a similar population. It is not known whether treatment of hypertension can prevent vascular dementia. In the same trial, in elderly people with isolated systolic hypertension, antihypertensive treatment was associated with a lower incidence of dementia (vascular but also Alzheimer's disease) [4]. Their findings suggested that if 1,000 hypertensive patients were treated with antihypertensive drugs for 5 years, 19 cases of dementia would be prevented. In the Study on Cognition and Prognosis in the Elderly, elderly patients with mildly to moderately elevated blood pressure, who received angiotensin receptor blocker candesartan-based therapy, had a slightly larger reduction in blood pressure than patients receiving placebo. This was associated with a modest, statistically nonsignificant reduction in major cardiovascular events and a marked reduction in nonfatal stroke. However, cognitive function was well maintained in both treatment groups in the presence of substantial reductions in blood pressure [5]. More recent analyses suggested that candesartan-based treatment improved cognitive function and quality of life in old and very old patients with mild to moderate hypertension [6, 7]. In the Rotterdam study, subjects taking antihypertensive medication at baseline (n = 2,015), who were then followed for a mean of 2.2 years, had a reduced incidence of dementia (adjusted relative risk, 0.76; 95% CI, 0.52–1.12). This reduction in risk was most pronounced for vascular dementia (adjusted relative risk, 0.30; 95% CI, 0.11–0.99) [8]. Thus, there seems to be clear prognostic benefits of treatment that lowers blood pressure in hypertensive patients.

Randomized controlled trials addressing interventions to minimize other risk factors mentioned above, such as warfarin treatment in atrial fibrillation or carotid endarterectomy, based their study end-points on the prevention of strokes and not the prevention of dementia. This is also true for the study of statins. Statins have been shown to prevent both incident and recurrent cerebral ischemic stroke [9–11]. Given the benefit of preventing recurrent stroke, it would seem reasonable to treat vascular dementia patients with statin therapy to prevent stroke. To date, however, there is no evidence that statin therapy reduces the risk of incident dementia. A post-hoc analysis of the Cardiovascular Health Study revealed a trend towards reduced cognitive decline in patients treated with statins, but there was no change in the risk of incident dementia in this cohort [12–13]. Similarly, two other prospective cohort studies also failed to show a reduction in dementia associated with statin use [14–15]. A large randomized controlled trial in Australia, the ASPirin in Reducing Events in the Elderly trial, is currently ongoing; this study is investigating the use of 100 mg of aspirin for the primary prevention of major adverse events and vascular dementia [16].

After Stroke or Silent Cerebral Ischemia (Secondary Prevention)
This deals with early management of acute stroke, preventing recurrent stroke and reducing the progression of vascular-related changes in the brain by treating vascular risk factors. The Perindopril Protection Against Recurrent Stroke Study [17] showed that active treatment by an angiotensin-converting enzyme inhibitor, used alone or combined with a diuretic, was associated with a reduced risk of dementia and cognitive decline in patients with recurrent stroke. In addition, an active blood pressure-lowering regimen stopped or delayed the progression of white matter hyperintensities detected on cerebral MRI in patients with cerebrovascular disease [18].

Curative Treatment

Once dementia has begun, new infarcts need to be prevented and its progression needs to be slowed down. A variety of treatments for vascular dementia have been tested. These include agents which affect cerebral blood flow. Meyer et al. [19] report encouraging results from a randomized clinical trial testing 325 mg of aspirin per day in 70 patients with vascular dementia. Daily aspirin treatment improved cognitive performance and reduced or stabilized the decline in cerebral perfusion in this group of patients. The authors stated that this treatment also improved quality of life and independence in daily activities. Nimodipine treatment has also been suggested for vascular dementia. This drug exerts its vasoactive effects by dilating mostly small and collateral cerebral vessels and improving blood supply to underperfused areas. In an open trial [20], cognitive function was found to stabilize in 31 patients treated with a daily dose of 90 mg nimodipine for up to 1 year. However, it is very difficult to draw any firm conclusions in the absence of randomized placebo-controlled studies of large populations. In a double-blind, placebo-controlled study [21], 112 patients were treated with nicergoline, a thrombolytic, vasoactive ergot alkaloid. Nicergoline improved vigilance and information processing in the neuropsychological assessment of patients with degenerative and vascular dementia. Several studies have investigated the use of pentoxifylline, which has been approved for use in peripheral vascular disease (intermittent claudication) and is reported to have a 'hemorheological' mode of action, i.e. it is thought to affect the microcirculation, increasing capillary blood flow and thereby improving tissue oxygenation [22, 23]. These studies suggested that the treatment may be beneficial but the differences between patients receiving treatment and those given the placebo were small and often not statistically significant. Another drug which may be effective is propentofylline [24–26], which strongly inhibits the potentially neurotoxic actions of activated microglia (free radical formation and transformation into brain macrophages). This drug may inhibit the progressive neurodegenerative process in dementia; however, randomized, double-blind placebo-controlled trials are required to establish whether this drug is effective. Long-term benefits have not been consistently demonstrated for any of these drugs. A recent Cochrane review (meta-analyses of 29 studies; total participants = 4,247) on *Ginkgo biloba* extract, concluded that the evidence that *Ginkgo* has predictable or clinically significant benefit for people with dementia (all etiologies) or cognitive impairment is inconsistent and unconvincing [27].

Recent evidence supports the involvement of the cholinergic system in vascular dementia, similar to that seen in Alzheimer's disease (AD). The mechanism of action of cholinesterase inhibitors in vascular dementia should, however, be investigated further [28, 29]. Several studies have tried to determine the effect of cholinesterase inhibitors on vascular dementia, but the results are also limited and inconsistent. A recent meta-analysis of randomized controlled trials concluded that cholinesterase inhibitors and memantine produce small benefits in cognitive function and do not necessarily have clinical significance in patients with mild to moderate vascular dementia [30]. According to the authors, there are insufficient data to support widespread use of these drugs in vascular dementia. The trials meeting the selection criteria for this meta-analysis included three donepezil (307, 308, 319) [31–33], two galantamine (GAL-INT-6 and 26) [34, 35], one rivastigmine (VantagE) [36], and two memantine trials (MMM300 and 500) [37, 38], comprising 3,093 patients on the study drugs and 2,090 patients on placebo (table 1). Cognitive effects on the Alzheimer's Disease Assessment Scale were significant for all drugs, ranging from a mean difference of –1.10 (95% CI –2.15 to –0.05) for rivastigmine to –2.17 for 10 mg daily donepezil (95% CI –2.98 to –1.35). Only 5 mg daily donepezil had an effect on the Clinicians' Global Impression of Change Scale [odds ratio 1.51 (95% CI 1.11–2.07)]. No behavioral or functional benefits were observed, except for a difference of –0.95 (95% CI –1.74 to –0.16) on the Alzheimer's Disease Functional Assessment and Change Scale for treatment with 10 mg daily donepezil. The main outcomes of these trials are described in table 2. Strengths of this meta-analysis include the exclusion of biased studies and the inclusion of unpublished results from three trials not included in previous reviews:

(1) The GAL-INT-26 study, which is now published, showed that galantamine was effective for improving cognition, including executive function, in patients with vascular dementia, with good safety and tolerability. However, improvement in

Table 1. Characteristics of patients from randomized controlled trials for cholinesterase inhibitors and memantine for vascular dementia

Trial	Design and patients							Characteristics of vascular lesions, %					
	Length weeks	Inclusion criteria [44–49]	Patients	Mean age	Males %	Mean MMSE	Mean ADAS-cog/11	Cortical only (single/multiple infarcts)[1]	Sub-cortical only (lacunes)[1]	Cortical and sub-cortical[1]	White matter only	Extensive white matter[1]	Combined with AD lesions
Donepezil 307 [31] 5 and 10 mg/day	24	probable or possible VaD [44] MD excluded	603	73.9 (7.37)	55	21.3 (4.25)	20.7 (10.4)	18–21	33–36	17–23	18	...	–
Donepezil 308 [32] 5 and 10 mg/day	24	probable or possible VaD [44] MD excluded	616	75.0 (7.44)	60	22.3 (4.31)	20.1 (10.0)	25	35	20	15	...	–
Donepezil 319 [33] 5 mg/day	24	probable or possible VaD [44] MD excluded	974	73.0 (9.36)	59	23.0 (–)	...	...	...	...	...	...	–
GAL-INT-6 [34] 24 mg/day	24	probable VaD [44] or MD [45]	592	75.1 (7.00)	53	20.5 (3.63)	22.8 (9.18)	39–46	40–47	7–8	...	64	48
GAL-INT-26 [35] 16 and 24 mg/day	26	probable VaD [44] MD excluded	788	72.3 (8.87)	64	20.3 (3.90)	22.7 (9.50)	41–46	31	...	...	52	–
VantagE [36] 6 to 12 mg/day	24	probable VaD [44, 46] MD excluded	710	72.9 (8.32)	61	19.2 (4.01)	23.3 (9.88)	...	...	...	...	69–72	–
MMM300 [37] 20 mg/day	28	probable VaD [44, 47] MD excluded	288	76.4 (6.68)	53	16.9 (2.52)	21.0 (9.15)	34–37	...	...	...	76–79	–
MMM500 [38] 20 mg/day	28	probable VaD [44, 48, 49] MD excluded	548	77.4 (6.94)	61	17.6 (3.25)	25.7 (11.0)	28–29	...	...	...	...	–

Figures in parentheses indicate SD. ... = Data not available; VaD = vascular dementia; AD = Alzheimer's disease; MMSE = Mini-Mental State Examination; ADAS-cog/11 = Alzheimer's Disease Assessment Scale-Cognitive subscale; mixed dementia = vascular dementia and Alzheimer's disease.
[1]Two results correspond to results in the treated and placebo groups respectively.

Table 2. Outcomes of randomized controlled trials for cholinesterase inhibitors and memantine for vascular dementia

Trial	Cognitive outcomes (ADAS-cog/MMSE)			Clinicians global outcomes (CGIC/CIBIC-plus)		Functional scales/behavior	
	treatment	placebo	comments	treatment	placebo	treatment vs. placebo	comments
Donepezil 307 [31] 5 and 10 mg/day	Improvement	Decline	Only 10 mg differed from placebo Post-hoc analyses suggested greater improvement in patients with cortical and multiple territorial lesions compared to those with predominantly subcortical lesions	Tendency to improve	No change	Not significant (ADFACS)	Only 5 mg was significantly associated with improvement or no change versus decline in global scores Only 10 mg differed from placebo in functional scales
Donepezil 308 [32] 5 and 10 mg/day	Improvement	Decline	Only 10 mg differed from placebo Post-hoc analyses suggested greater improvement in patients with cortical and multiple territorial lesions compared to those with predominantly subcortical lesions	Tendency to improve	No change	Not significant (ADFACS)	Only 5 mg was significantly associated with improvement or no change versus decline in global scores Only 10 mg differed from placebo in functional scales
Donepezil 319 [33] 5 mg/day	Tendency to improve	No change	Additional tests of frontal executive function did not improve detection of treatment effects	...	...	No significant (disability assessment for dementia)	
GAL-INT-6 [34] 24 mg/day	VaD: improvement MD: slight improvement	VaD: improvement MD: slight improvement		All cohort: improvement VaD: no change	No change	No significant (disability assessment for dementia; NPI)	
GAL-INT-26 [35] 16 and 24 mg/day	Improvement	No change	Post-hoc analyses suggested greater improvement in patients with cortical and multiple territorial lesions compared to those with predominantly subcortical lesions	Tendency to improve	No change	No significant (ADCS-ADL; NPI)	Post-hoc analyses suggested greater improvement in patients with cortical and multiple territorial lesions compared to those with predominantly subcortical lesions

Table 2. Continued

Trial	Cognitive outcomes (ADAS-cog/MMSE)			Clinicians global outcomes (CGIC/CIBIC-plus)		Functional scales/behavior	
	treatment	placebo	comments	treatment	placebo	treatment vs. placebo	comments
VantagE [36] 6 to 12 mg/day	Slight improvement	Slight decline	Additional tests of frontal executive function did not improve detection of treatment effects	Slight decline	Slight decline	No significant (ADCS-ADL; NPI)	
MMM300 [37] 20 mg/day	No change	No change	Larger effects in subgroups that predominantly had small vessel disease, and with MMSE<15, due to decline in placebo group	No change or tendency to improve	No change	No significant (NOSGER)	
MMM500 [38] 20 mg/day	No change	No change	Larger effects in subgroups who predominantly had small-vessel disease, and with MMSE<15, due to worsening in placebo group	...	...	No significant (NOSGER)	

... = Data not available; MD = mixed dementia (VaD and AD); ADAS-cog/11 = Alzheimer's Disease Assessment Scale-Cognitive subscale; CGIC = clinician's global impression of change; CIBIC-plus = clinicians' interview-based impression of change with caregiver's input; ADFACS = AD functional assessment and change; ADCS-ADL = AD Cooperative Study ADL inventory; NPI = Neuropsychiatric Inventory; NOSGER = Nurses' Observation Scale for Geriatric Patients.

performing daily activities in patients on galantamine was similar to that observed in patients receiving placebo [35].

(2) The VantagE study, which is now published, showed that rivastigmine was not consistently effective in probable vascular dementia. The efficacy in terms of cognitive outcome was based on effects in older patients likely to have concomitant AD pathology. This is consistent with previous findings suggesting that the putative cholinergic deficit in vascular dementia probably reflects the presence of concomitant AD pathology [36].

(3) The Donepezil 319 study remains unpublished [33].

The findings of this recent meta-analysis are not inconsistent with earlier reviews of rivastigmine, galantamine and memantine. Previous Cochrane reviews have concluded that there was insufficient evidence to support the use of these three drugs (galantamine, rivastigmine and memantine) in patients with vascular dementia [39–41]. However, results in the meta-analysis for donepezil differ from an earlier review of the Cochrane Database [42] and from a manufacturer-sponsored review [43]. This is mainly due to the inclusion of the unpublished trial (trial 319), which substantially attenuated the global effects observed for the 5 mg dose [from –0.24 (95% CI –0.40 to –0.08) to –0.15 (95% CI –0.26 to –0.04)]. At the same time, the risk of death was significantly higher with donepezil than with placebo in trial 319. The evidence of a smaller effect size for cognitive and global outcome, the suggestion of increased mortality with 5 mg donepezil, and the lack of overall benefit with the 10 mg dose, suggest that a guarded position on the use of donepezil for vascular dementia should be adopted.

Currently, there is not enough evidence to recommend cholinesterase inhibitors and memantine as treatment for vascular dementia. Regulatory approval for the treatment of vascular dementia with these drugs has not been acquired in most parts of the world, despite some positive but small effects observed in clinical trials.

Several important factors should be considered for the interpretation of clinical trials for vascular dementia:

The Heterogeneity of the Disease Itself

The trials included patients with clinically heterogeneous cerebrovascular disease and by design could not address whether particular patient subgroups might have benefited. Patients with vascular dementia varied widely in terms of type, location, and extent of cerebrovascular disease. Divergent processes (e.g. single large-vessel lesion or multiple infarct, diffuse leukoencephalopathy and/or lacunes) are potentially included and clinical presentation and progression may differ, and may respond differently to the drugs tested. Additional heterogeneity both within and between trials may result from different choices of diagnostic imaging methods. For example, trials relying to a greater degree on MRI than CT scans may have been more likely to identify patients with smaller lesions and white matter disease (table 1). Consequently, individual patient analyses are needed to identify subgroups of patients with vascular dementia who might benefit from a treatment.

The High Prevalence of Mixed Pathology, Especially in the Elderly

Vascular lesions coexisting with AD lesions may lead to the detection of small effects in the vascular dementia trials, due to effects on comorbid AD, specific subtypes of vascular dementia, or a combination of both.

Selection of Tools Specific to Vascular Pathology

The ADAS-cog test, used in AD trials, essentially provides a composite score of memory, language and orientation. It does not assess attention and the range of executive dysfunction or subcortical impairment associated with vascular dementia.

The Trial Length

The trials lasted 6 months and were designed to specifically assess symptomatic rather than neuroprotective effects.

Symptomatic Treatment of Cognitive and Neurological Deficits and the Support of Carers

Physiotherapy can avoid complications of motor function (scarring, ankyloses and retraction of the tendons), increasing the patient's level of independence. Speech therapy is also beneficial. Rehabilitation is often limited by progression of the dementia. At this stage of the illness, simple practical measures such as avoiding falls are very effective. It is also of utmost importance to ensure that the drug treatment does not provoke hypotension.

In general, the management of patients with vascular dementia is similar to that of other dementia patients. If possible, the patient is cared for at home, isolation of the subject is avoided and close attention is paid to the prescription of drugs. Behavioral problems, secondary depression, intercurrent affections and metabolic problems are treated and the patient is made a ward of court if necessary. Family support is encouraged and most importantly, the patient's future is considered.

Conclusions

Vascular dementia is potentially preventable by treating risk factors very early in midlife. It is vital to reduce all cerebrovascular risks, especially hypertension. Curative treatment of vascular dementia is still ineffective, although a number of drugs are currently under investigation. Well-designed and adequately powered trials that account for the heterogeneity of vascular dementia are needed. These trials should use optimal clinical definitions (stratifying by pathology/mechanisms for example) and more specific tools for the detection of cognitive and global changes in vascular dementia. They should allow for the extensive post-hoc analyses required in patients with significant medical and psychiatric comorbidity. The support of carers in the patient's family is essential if elderly patients are to be cared for in the community. This involves assessing the social integration, occupational activity, leisure activity, economic problems and family conflicts associated with sharing the responsibility of caring. By focusing on these aspects we should be able to develop successful intervention strategies to treat vascular dementia.

References

1 Whitmer RA, Sidney S, Selby J, Claiborne Johnston S, Yaffe K: Midlife cardiovascular risk factors and risk of dementia in late life. Neurology 2005;64:277–281.

2 SHEP Cooperative Research Group: Prevention of stroke by antihypertensive drug treatment in older persons with isolated systolic hypertension. J Am Med Assoc 1991;265:3225–3264.

3 Staessen JA, Fagard R, Thijs L, Celis H, Arabidze GG, Birkenhäger WH, Bulpitt CJ, de Leeuw PW, Dollery CT, Fletcher AE, Forette F, Leonetti G, Nachev C, O'Brien ET, Rosenfeld J, Rodicio JL, Tuomilehto J, Zanchetti A: Randomized double-blind comparison of placebo and active treatment of older patients with isolated systolic hypertension. Lancet 1997;350:757–764.

4 Forette F, Seux ML, Staessen JA Thijs L, Birkenhäger WH, Babarskiene MR, Babeanu S, Bossini A, Gil-Extremera B, Girerd X, Laks T, Lilov E, Moisseyev V, Tuomilehto J, Vanhanen H, Webster J, Yodfat Y, Fagard R: Prevention of dementia in randomised double-blind placebo-controlled Systolic Hypertension in Europe (Syst-Eur) trial. Lancet 1998;24; 352: 1347–1351.

5 Lithell H, Hansson L, Skoog I, Elmfeldt D, Hofman A, Olofsson B, Trenkwalder P, Zanchetti A, SCOPE Study Group: The Study on Cognition and Prognosis in the Elderly (SCOPE): principal results of a randomized double-blind intervention trial. J Hypertens 2003;21:875–886.

6 Trenkwalder P: The Study on COgnition and Prognosis in the Elderly (SCOPE) – recent analyses. J Hypertens Suppl 2006;24:S107—S114.

7 Zanchetti A, Elmfeldt D: Findings and implications of the Study on COgnition and Prognosis in the Elderly (SCOPE) – a review. Blood Press 2006;15:71–79.

8 in t' Veld BA, Ruitenberg A, Hofman A, Stricker BH, Breteler MM: Antihypertensive drugs and incidence of dementia: the Rotterdam Study. Neurobiol Aging 2001;22:407–412.

9 Amarenco P, Bogousslavsky J, Callahan A 3rd, Goldstein LB, Hennerici M, Rudolph AE, Sillesen H, Simunovic L, Szarek M, Welch KM, Zivin JA, Stroke Prevention by Aggressive Reduction in Cholesterol Levels (SPARCL) Investigators: High-dose atorvastatin after stroke or transient ischemic attack. N Engl J Med 2006;355:549–559.

10 MRC/BHF Heart Protection Study of cholesterol lowering with simvastatin in 20,536 high-risk individuals: a randomised placebo-controlled trial. Lancet 2002;360:7–22.

11 Shepherd J, Blauw GJ, Murphy MB, Bollen EL, Buckley BM, Cobbe SM, Ford I, Gaw A, Hyland M, Jukema JW, Kamper AM, Macfarlane PW, Meinders AE, Norrie J, Packard CJ, Perry IJ, Stott DJ, Sweeney BJ, Twomey C, Westendorp RG, PROSPER study group: PROspective Study of Pravastatin in the Elderly at Risk. Pravastatin in elderly individuals at risk of vascular disease (PROSPER): a randomised controlled trial. Lancet. 2002;360:1623–1630.

12 Bernick C, Katz R, Smith NL, Rapp S, Bhadelia R, Carlson M, Kuller L, Cardiovascular Health Study Collaborative Research Group: Statins and cognitive function in the elderly: the Cardiovascular Health Study. Neurology 2005;65:1388–1394.

13 Rea TD, Breitner JC, Psaty BM, Fitzpatrick AL, Lopez OL, Newman AB, Hazzard WR, Zandi PP, Burke GL, Lyketsos CG, Bernick C, Kuller LH: Statin use and the risk of incident dementia: the Cardiovascular Health Study. Arch Neurol 2005; 62:1047–1051.

14 Li G, Higdon R, Kukull WA, Peskind E, Van Valen Moore K, Tsuang D, van Belle G, McCormick W, Bowen JD, Teri L, Schellenberg GD, Larson EB: Statin therapy and risk of dementia in the elderly: a community-based prospective cohort study. Neurology 2004;63:1624–1628.

15 Zandi PP, Sparks DL, Khachaturian AS, Tschanz J, Norton M, Steinberg M, Welsh-Bohmer KA, Breitner JC, Cache County Study investigators: Do statins reduce risk of incident dementia and Alzheimer disease? The Cache County Study. Arch Gen Psychiatry 2005;62:217–224.

16 Nelson MR, Reid CM, Ames DA, Beilin LJ, Donnan GA, Gibbs P, Johnston CI, Krum H, Storey E, Tonkin A, Wolfe R, Woods R, McNeil JJ: Feasibility of conducting a primary prevention trial of low-dose aspirin for major adverse cardiovascular events in older people in Australia: results from the ASPirin in Reducing Events in the Elderly (ASPREE) pilot study. Med J Aust 2008;189:105–109.

17 Tzourio C, Anderson C, Chapman N, Woodward M, Neal B, MacMahon S, Chalmers J, PROGRESS Collaborative Group: Effects of blood pressure lowering with perindopril and indapamide therapy on dementia and cognitive decline in patients with cerebrovascular disease. Arch Intern Med 2003;163:1069–1075.

18 Dufouil C, Chalmers J, Coskun O, Besançon V, Bousser MG, Guillon P, MacMahon S, Mazoyer B, Neal B, Woodward M, Tzourio-Mazoyer N, Tzourio C, PROGRESS MRI Substudy Investigators: Effects of blood pressure lowering on cerebral white matter hyperintensities in patients with stroke: the PROGRESS (Perindopril Protection Against Recurrent Stroke Study) Magnetic Resonance Imaging Substudy. Circulation 2005;112:1644–1650.

19 Meyer JS, Rogers RL, McClintic K, Mortel KF, Lotfi J: Randomized clinical trial of daily aspirin therapy in multi-infarct dementia: a pilot study. J Am Geriatr Soc 1989;37:549–555.

20 Pantoni L, Carosi M, Amigoni S, Mascalchi M, Inzitari D: A preliminary open trial with nimodipine in patients with cognitive impairment and leukoaraiosis. Clin Neuropharmacol 1996;19:497–506.

21 Saletu B, Paulus E, Linzmayer L, Anderer P, Semlitsch HV, Grunberger J, Wicke L, Neuhold A, Podreka I: Nicergoline in senile dementia of Alzheimer type and multi-infarct dementia: a double-bind, placebo-controlled, clinical and EEG/ERP mapping study. Psychopharmacology 1995;117:385–395.
22 Black RS, Barclay LL, Nolan KA, Thaler HT, Hardiman ST, Blass JP: Pentoxifylline in cerebrovascular dementia. J Am Geriatr Soc 1992;40:237–244.
23 European Pentoxifylline Multi-infarct Dementia Study. Eur Neurol 1996;36:315–321.
24 Huber M, Kittner B, Hojer C, Fink GR, Neveling M, Heiss WD: Effect of propentofylline on regional cerebral glucose metabolism in acute ischemic stroke. J Cereb Blood Flow Metab 1993;13:526–530.
25 Kittner B, Rossner M, Rother M: Clinical trials in dementia with propentofylline. Ann N Y Acad Sci 1997;826:307–316.
26 Marcusson J, Rother M, Kittner B, Rossner M, Smith RJ, Babic T, Folnegovic-Smalc V, Moller HJ, Labs KH: A 12-month, randomized, placebo-controlled trial of propentofylline (HWA 285) in patients with dementia according to DSM III-R. The European Propentofylline Study Group. Dement Geriatr Cogn Disord 1997;8:320–328.
27 Birks J, Grimley Evans J: Ginkgo biloba for cognitive impairment and dementia. Cochrane Database Syst Rev 2007:CD003120.
28 Grantham C, Geerts H: The rationale behind cholinergic drug treatment for dementia related to cerebrovascular disease. J Neurol Sci 2002;203:131–136.
29 Roman G, Kalaria R: Vascular determinants of cholinergic deficits in Alzheimer disease and vascular dementia. Neurobiol Aging 2006;27:1769–1785.
30 Kavirajan H, Schneider LS: Efficacy and adverse effects of cholinesterase inhibitors and memantine in vascular dementia: a meta-analysis of randomised controlled trials. Lancet Neurol 2007;6:782–792.
31 Black S, Roman GC, Geldmacher DS, Salloway S, Hecker J, Burns A, Perdomo C, Kumar D, Pratt R, Donepezil 307 Vascular Dementia Study Group: Efficacy and tolerability of donepezil in vascular dementia: positive results of a 24-week, multicenter, international, randomized, placebo-controlled clinical trial. Stroke 2003;34:2323–2330.
32 Wilkinson D, Doody R, Helme R, Taubman K, Mintzer J, Kertesz A, Pratt RD, Donepezil 308 Study Group: Donepezil in vascular dementia: a randomized, placebo-controlled study. Neurology 2003;61:479–486.
33 Eisai Co Ltd News Release: Eisai reports results from latest donepezil study in vascular dementia http://www.eisai.co.jp/enews/enews200609.html (March 16, 2006).
34 Erkinjuntti T, Kurz A, Gauthier S, Bullock R, Lilienfeld S, Damaraju CV: Efficacy of galantamine in probable vascular dementia and Alzheimer's disease combined with cerebrovascular disease: a randomised trial. Lancet 2002;359:1283–1290.
35 Auchus AP, Brashear HR, Salloway S, Korczyn AD, De Deyn PP, Gassmann-Mayer C, GAL-INT-26 Study Group: Galantamine treatment of vascular dementia: a randomized trial. Neurology 2007;69:448–458.
36 Ballard C, Sauter M, Scheltens P, He Y, Barkhof F, van Straaten EC, van der Flier WM, Hsu C, Wu S, Lane R: Efficacy, safety and tolerability of rivastigmine capsules in patients with probable vascular dementia: the VantagE study. Curr Med Res Opin 2008;24:2564–2574.
37 Orgogozo JM, Rigaud AS, Stöffler A, Möbius HJ, Forette F: Efficacy and safety of memantine in patients with mild to moderate vascular dementia: a randomized, placebo-controlled trial (MMM 300). Stroke 2002;33:1834–1839.
38 Wilcock G, Mobius HJ, Stoffler A: A double-blind, placebo-controlled multicentre study of memantine in mild to moderate vascular dementia (MMM500). Int Clin Psychopharmacol 2002;17:297–305.
39 Craig D, Birks J: Galantamine for vascular cognitive impairment. Cochrane Database Syst Rev 2006: CD004746.
40 Craig D, Birks J: Rivastigmine for vascular cognitive impairment. Cochrane Database Syst Rev 2005: CD004744.
41 McShane R, Areosa Sastre A, Minakaran N: Memantine for dementia. Cochrane Database Syst Rev 2006:CD003154.
42 Malouf R, Birks J: Donepezil for vascular cognitive impairment. Cochrane Database Syst Rev 2004: CD004395.
43 Roman G, Wilkinson D, Doody R, Black S, Salloway S, Schindler R: Donepezil in vascular dementia: combined analysis of two large-scale clinical trials. Dement Geriatr Cogn Disord 2005;20:338–344.
44 Román GC, Tatemichi TK, Erkinjuntti T, Cummings JL, Masdeu JC, Garcia JH, Amaducci L, Orgogozo JM, Brun A, Hofman A, et al: Vascular dementia: diagnostic criteria for research studies: report of the NINDS-AIREN International Workshop. Neurology 1993;43:250–260.
45 McKahn G, Drachman D, Folstein M, Katzman R, Price D, Stadlan EM: Clinical diagnosis of Alzheimer's disease: report of the NINCDS-ADRDA Work Group under the auspices of the Department of Health and Human Services Task Force on Alzheimer's Disease. Neurology 1984;34:939–944.

46 American Psychiatry Association: Diagnostic and Statistical Manual of Mental Disorders, ed 4. Washington, American Psychiatry Association, 1994, pp 143–146.
47 Rosen WG, Terry R, Fuld A, Katzman R, Peck A: Pathological verification verification of ischemic score in differentiation of dementias. Ann Neurol 1980;7:486–488.
48 American Psychiatry Association: Diagnostic and Statistical Manual of Mental Disorders, DSM-III-R. Washington, American Psychiatry Association, 1987.
49 Hachinski VC, Iliff LD, Zilhka E, Du Boulay GHD, McAllister VL, Marshall J, Russel RWR, Symon L: Cerebral blood flow in dementia. Arch Neurol 1975;32:632–637.

Dr. Dina Zekry
Hôpital des Trois-Chênes
3, chemin du Pont-Bochet
CH–1226 Thônex, Geneva (Switzerland)
Tel. +41 22 305 6355, Fax +41 22 305 6115, E-Mail Dina.Zekry@hcuge.ch

Giannakopoulos P, Hof PR (eds): Dementia in Clinical Practice.
Front Neurol Neurosci. Basel, Karger, 2009, vol 24, pp 107–113

Dementia with Lewy Bodies: Clinical Diagnosis and Therapeutic Approach

Gabriel Gold

Geneva University School of Medicine and Geneva University Hospitals, Geneva, Switzerland

Abstract

Dementia with Lewy bodies is one of the most common dementias in the elderly after Alzheimer's disease. It can be recognized on the basis of several clinical characteristics including progressive dementia with marked slowing and fluctuations, persistent visual hallucinations and an extrapyramidal syndrome. Several other clinical and imaging features are highly suggestive such as the presence of rapid eye movement sleep disorder, severe sensitivity to neuroleptics and specific neuroimaging abnormalities. Therapeutic strategies include prescription of L-dopa and cholinesterase inhibitors such as rivastigmine, and avoidance of anticholinergic medications and neuroleptics. Physicians who care for older people should have a heightened awareness of this entity in order to diagnose it early, avoid mistaking it for delirium and initiate appropriate treatment.

In 1912, Friedrich Lewy described inclusion bodies that now bear his name in the substantia nigra of patients presenting with 'paralysis agitans'. In 1961, Okazaki described Lewy bodies in the cortex of patients with cognitive impairment. At the end of the 20th century, dementia with Lewy bodies (DLB) was finally recognized as a specific and different type of dementia. Since then, progress in the identification of the clinical characteristics of DLB and improved neuropathological staining methods have led to a greater recognition of DLB as one of the most common dementias in older populations occurring in 10–20% of pathological series [1].

Clinical Presentation and Diagnostic Clues

Many clinicians who are familiar with Alzheimer's disease (AD) and vascular dementia, the two most common causes of dementia in the elderly, may experience difficulty in recognizing DLB. It is important to note that several clinical features are highly suggestive of this diagnosis. In particular, DLB should be strongly suspected in individuals who present with the following triad: dementia, visual hallucinations and an extrapyramidal syndrome.

Dementia with Fluctuating Cognition

The cognitive dysfunction is usually of insidious onset and affects memory and other domains. Clues to the presence of DLB include slowing and marked fluctuations in attention and cognitive performance. The fluctuations are striking, and sometimes difficult to distinguish from a delirium, particularly since changes in attention are often accompanied by daytime sleepiness and impaired level of consciousness [2]. This can be problematic since some of the medications used for the treatment of delirium are contraindicated in the presence of DLB. The general pattern of cognitive deficits in DLB is detailed below (see 'Neuropsychological Profile', below) but it is important to remember that results of psychometric evaluations tend to vary due not only to changes in attention but also to periods of highly disorganized and illogical thinking.

Extrapyramidal Syndrome

Dementia and the extrapyramidal syndrome usually present within the same year. The extrapyramidal syndrome is generally of moderate intensity and often symmetrical, tremor is usually not prominent and atypical; response to L-dopa is generally modest. However, it is important to remember that none of the symptoms of the associated extrapyramidal syndrome are characteristic of DLB.

Hallucinations

Visual hallucinations are reported in 80% of the cases. They are persistent and must be distinguished from hallucinations that may occur transiently upon introduction or dose modification of therapy for the associated extrapyramidal syndrome. Patients usually recognize that the hallucinations are not real and often do not report them spontaneously. Auditory hallucinations may also occur but they are less common.

Several other clinical features are also suggestive of DLB.

Severe Neuroleptic Sensitivity

Adverse reactions to neuroleptics include severe extrapyramidal symptoms, altered consciousness and increased confusion. This clinical feature was recognized quite early as a highly suggestive clue to the presence of DLB; however, it occurs in approximately half of the cases only [3, 4]. Furthermore, complications can be serious; therefore, prescribing neuroleptics as a diagnostic test is not recommended.

Rapid Eye Movement Sleep Behavior Disorder

Rapid eye movement (REM) sleep is accompanied by muscle atonia preventing individuals from acting out their dreams. In DLB, muscle activity can occur during REM sleep resulting at times in complex movements. The spouse or care giving staff may report agitated sleep, vivid dreams or a chaotic state of the bedcovers in the morning. This finding is highly suggestive of neurodegenerative disease involving α-synuclein such as DLB, Parkinson's disease and multisystem atrophy [5–7]. It may be one of the earliest signs of such pathology and has been reported to precede other symptoms by as much as 20 years [8]. In unclear cases, polysomnography can be used to document REM sleep without atonia.

Neuropsychological Profile

The neuropsychological evaluation can identify impairments that are consistent with DLB but, more importantly, it can provide key information to help distinguish this entity from AD [for reviews, see 9, 10].

The memory deficit is mild and relatively stable initially as opposed to AD where it is the central feature. Working and semantic memory are affected similarly in both entities [10]. Verbal tests of episodic memory show greater decline in AD but visual memory tests show no difference between DLB and AD [9–12].

Visuospatial skills are affected early in DLB, and copying performance is usually worse than in AD cases of comparable severity. This can be demonstrated with relatively simple tasks such as copying a cube or interlocking pentagons [13]. In general, AD patients tend to have difficulty copying from memory whereas DLB patients encounter difficulty secondary to impaired perception and praxia [10]. In a comparison of 10 DLB and 9 AD patients matched for age, education and global dementia severity (as measured by the Mini-Mental State Examination), performance on the Visual Object and Space Perception Test demonstrated substantial impairments in object and space perception in the DLB group but not in the AD cases [14]. In another study, individuals with DLB had greater deficits in visual discrimination, object perception and space motion tasks compared with AD cases [15].

Attention and executive function including visual attention, ability to suppress distraction, shifting mental sets and initiation appear to be more severely impaired in DLB.

Neuroimaging Data

Structural neuroimaging such as CT or MRI can help rule out vascular pathology but does not clearly differentiate DLB from AD and normal aging [16]. Although medial temporal atrophy is more common in AD, it can also occur in half or more of DLB cases [17–18].

Several single photon emission computed tomography (SPECT) studies have reported decreased occipital perfusion in DLB especially when compared with AD [19–21]. However, a recent study found similar rates of occipital hypoperfusion in

DLB (28%) and non-DLB (31%) patients [22]. Fluorodeoxyglucose positron emission tomography reveals occipital hypometabolism in DLB and may perform better than SPECT in differentiating this entity from AD, but most studies include small numbers of patients and retrospectively determined thresholds [16].

Bilateral reduction in medial temporal perfusion is described in AD and consistent with hippocampal involvement in this disease; however, medial temporal hypoperfusion can also occur in DLB. Many studies have compared the frequency of this finding in AD and DLB with conflicting results [19, 23–25]. Parietotemporal hypoperfusion and hypometabolism are a well-described finding in AD; however, it has also been described in DLB and cannot be reliably used to distinguish these two types of dementia [16, 26–27].

Several ligands have been developed for SPECT and PET imaging of presynaptic dopamine transporters [16] that can be used to visualize the loss of presynaptic dopaminergic neurons to the putamen and globus pallidus in DLB. This methodology has been found to be highly accurate when autopsy findings are used as a gold standard. In a series of 20 cases that underwent such scanning ante-mortem, the sensitivity and specificity for DLB were 88 and 100% compared with 75 and 42% for clinical criteria [25, 28]. Imaging of postsynaptic dopaminergic D2 receptors has shown an increase in the putamen and decrease in the caudate in DLB compared with AD; unfortunately, the important overlap between both groups markedly limits the diagnostic use of this imaging technique for individual cases [29].

Clinical Criteria

The consortium on DLB has produced diagnostic criteria based on the above findings. The latest revised version was published in 2005 [30]. It includes a required central feature (dementia), core features, suggestive features and supportive features. The latter have no proven diagnostic specificity and are not particularly useful for clinicians; the first three types of features are detailed in table 1.

Therapeutic Options

Adverse reactions and increased sensitivity to neuroleptics have been described with traditional as well as some atypical neuroleptics [3, 31]. Thus, such medications should be avoided whenever possible. If absolutely necessary, it should be kept in mind that both olanzapine and quetiapine have been used safely in cases with DLB and have led to a reduction in behavioral and psychiatric symptoms in studies with a small number of subjects [32, 33]. However, a recent trial of quetiapine that included 40 patients with DLB confirmed the good tolerance of the drug but did not show any benefit on agitation and psychosis compared with placebo [34].

Table 1. Central, core, and suggestive features of the revised criteria for the clinical diagnosis of DLB

1. Central features (essential for a diagnosis of possible or probable DLB) Dementia defined as progressive cognitive decline of sufficient magnitude to interfere with normal social or occupational function Prominent or persistent memory impairment may not necessarily occur in the early stages but is usually evident with progression Deficits on tests of attention, executive function, and visuospatial ability may be especially prominent
2. Core features (two core features are sufficient for a diagnosis of probable DLB or one for possible DLB) Fluctuating cognition with pronounced variations in attention and alertness Recurrent visual hallucinations that are typically well formed and detailed Spontaneous features of parkinsonism
3. Suggestive features (if one or more of these is present in the presence of one or more core features, a diagnosis of probable DLB can be made; in the absence of any core features, one or more suggestive features are sufficient for possible DLB; probable DLB should not be diagnosed on the basis of suggestive features alone) REM sleep behavior disorder Severe neuroleptic sensitivity Low dopamine transporter uptake in the basal ganglia demonstrated by SPECT or PET imaging

Adapted with permission from Mc Keith et al. [30].

DLB is associated with a cerebral cholinergic deficit [35]. As a result, drugs with anticholinergic side effects should be avoided. Trials of anticholinesterase inhibitors have generally been positive but often of small size [36, 37]. A larger trial of 120 patients with DLB showed significant benefits of rivastigmine on behavior and attention tasks and processing speed [38].

The extrapyramidal syndrome of DLB can be treated with levodopa [30]. The latter should be introduced at low doses and slowly increased to avoid initiating or exacerbating psychotic symptoms. Anticholinergic therapy of extrapyramidal symptoms should be avoided.

Conclusions

DLB is a common cause of dementia in the elderly. It is characterized by marked fluctuations in attention and cognitive function that can mimic delirium and lead to erroneous and possible dangerous prescription of neuroleptics. However, awareness of simple diagnostic clues can greatly facilitate early diagnosis and initiation of appropriate therapy. Recent advances in neuroimaging of presynaptic dopamine transporters can greatly enhance diagnostic accuracy and have been included in revised diagnostic criteria. Further research should focus on the development of therapeutic interventions which currently remain modestly effective.

References

1 McKeith I, Mintzer J, Aarsland D, Burn D, Chiu H, Cohen-Mansfield J, Dickson D, Dubois B, Duda JE, Feldman H, Gauthier S, Halliday G, Lawlor B, Lippa C, Lopez OL, Carlos Machado J, O'Brien J, Playfer J, Reid W: Dementia with Lewy bodies. Lancet Neurol 2004;3:19–28.

2 Ferman TJ, Smith GE, Boeve BF, Ivnik RJ, Petersen RC, Knopman D, Graff-Radford N, Parisi J, Dickson DW: DLB fluctuations: specific features that reliably differentiate DLB from AD and normal aging. Neurology 2004;62:181–187.

3 McKeith I, Fairbairn A, Perry R, Thompson P, Perry E: Neuroleptic sensitivity in patients with senile dementia of Lewy body type. Br Med J 1992;305: 673–678.

4 Ballard C, Grace J, McKeith I, Holmes C: Neuroleptic sensitivity in dementia with Lewy bodies and Alzheimer's disease. Lancet 1998;351:1032–1033.

5 Plazzi G, Corsini R, Provini F, Pierangeli G, Martinelli P, Montagna P, Lugaresi E, Cortelli P: REM sleep behavior disorders in multiple system atrophy. Neurology 1997;48:1094–1097.

6 Gagnon JF, Bedard MA, Fantini ML, Petit D, Panisset M, Rompre S, Carrier J, Montplaisir J: REM sleep behavior disorder and REM sleep without atonia in Parkinson's disease. Neurology 2002;59:585–589.

7 Turner RS, Chervin RD, Frey KA, Minoshima S, Kuhl DE: Probable diffuse Lewy body disease presenting as REM sleep behavior disorder. Neurology 1997;49:523–527.

8 Uchiyama M, Isse K, Tanaka K, Yokota N, Hamamoto M, Aida S, Ito Y, Yoshimura M, Okawa M: Incidental Lewy body disease in a patient with REM sleep behavior disorder. Neurology 1995;45: 709–712.

9 Collerton D, Burn D, McKeith I, O'Brien J: Systematic review and meta-analysis show that dementia with Lewy bodies is a visual-perceptual and attentional-executive dementia. Dement Geriatr Cogn Disord 2003;16:229–237.

10 Metzler-Baddeley C: A review of cognitive impairments in dementia with Lewy bodies relative to Alzheimer's disease and Parkinson's disease with dementia. Cortex 2007;43:583–600.

11 Simard M, van Reekum R, Cohen T: A review of the cognitive and behavioral symptoms in dementia with Lewy bodies. J Neuropsychiatry Clin Neurosci 2000;12:425–450.

12 Noe E, Marder K, Bell KL, Jacobs DM, Manly JJ, Stern Y: Comparison of dementia with Lewy bodies to Alzheimer's disease and Parkinson's disease with dementia. Mov Disord 2004;19:60–67.

13 Cormack F, Aarsland D, Ballard C, Tovee MJ: Pentagon drawing and neuropsychological performance in dementia with Lewy bodies, Alzheimer's disease, Parkinson's disease and Parkinson's disease with dementia. Int J Geriatr Psychiatry 2004;19:371–377.

14 Calderon J, Perry RJ, Erzinclioglu SW, Berrios GE, Dening TR, Hodges JR: Perception, attention, and working memory are disproportionately impaired in dementia with Lewy bodies compared with Alzheimer's disease. J Neurol Neurosurg Psychiatry 2001;70:157–164.

15 Mosimann UP, Mather G, Wesnes KA, O'Brien JT, Burn DJ, McKeith IG: Visual perception in Parkinson disease dementia and dementia with Lewy bodies. Neurology 2004;63:2091–2096.

16 Kemp PM, Holmes C: Imaging in dementia with Lewy bodies: a review. Nucl Med Commun 2007; 28:511–519.

17 Barber R, Gholkar A, Scheltens P, Ballard C, McKeith IG, O'Brien JT: Medial temporal lobe atrophy on MRI in dementia with Lewy bodies. Neurology 1999; 52:1153–1158.

18 Pasquier F, Hamon M, Lebert F, Jacob B, Pruvo JP, Petit H: Medial temporal lobe atrophy in memory disorders. J Neurol 1997;244:175–181.

19 Colloby SJ, Fenwick JD, Williams ED, Paling SM, Lobotesis K, Ballard C, McKeith I, O'Brien JT: A comparison of 99mTC-HMPAO SPECT changes in dementia with Lewy bodies and Alzheimer's disease using statistical parametric mapping. Eur J Nucl Med Mol Imaging 2002;29:615–622.

20 Lobotesis K, Fenwick JD, Phipps A, Ryman A, Swann A, Ballard C, McKeith IG, O'Brien JT: Occipital hypoperfusion on SPECT in dementia with Lewy bodies but not AD. Neurology 2001;56: 643–649.

21 Hanyu H, Shimizu S, Hirao K, Kanetaka H, Iwamoto T, Chikamori T, Usui Y, Yamashina A, Koizumi K, Abe K: Comparative value of brain perfusion SPECT and [(123)I]MIBG myocardial scintigraphy in distinguishing between dementia with Lewy bodies and Alzheimer's disease. Eur J Nucl Med Mol Imaging 2006;33:248–253.
22 Kemp PM, Hoffmann SA, Tossici-Bolt L, Fleming JS, Holmes C: Limitations of the HMPAO SPECT appearances of occipital lobe perfusion in the differential diagnosis of dementia with Lewy bodies. Nucl Med Commun 2007;28:451–456.
23 Minoshima S, Foster NL, Sima AA, Frey KA, Albin RL, Kuhl DE: Alzheimer's disease versus dementia with Lewy bodies: cerebral metabolic distinction with autopsy confirmation. Ann Neurol 2001;50: 358–365.
24 Higuchi M, Tashiro M, Arai H, Okamura N, Hara S, Higuchi S, Itoh M, Shin RW, Trojanowski JQ, Sasaki H: Glucose hypometabolism and neuropathological correlates in brains of dementia with Lewy bodies. Exp Neurol 2000;162:247–256.
25 Imamura T, Ishii K, Sasaki M, Kitagaki H, Yamaji S, Hirono N, Shimomura T, Hashimoto M, Tanimukai S, Kazui H, Mori E: Regional cerebral glucose metabolism in dementia with Lewy bodies and Alzheimer's disease: a comparative study using positron emission tomography. Neurosci Lett 1997;235: 49–52.
26 Pasquier J, Michel BF, Brenot-Rossi I, Hassan-Sebbag N, Sauvan R, Gastaut JL: Value of 99mTc-ECD SPECT for the diagnosis of dementia with Lewy bodies. Eur J Nucl Med Mol Imaging 2002;29: 1342–1348.
27 Shimizu S, Hanyu H, Kanetaka H, Iwamoto T, Koizumi K, Abe K: Differentiation of dementia with Lewy bodies from Alzheimer's disease using brain SPECT. Dement Geriatr Cogn Disord 2005;20:25–30.
28 Walker Z, Jaros E, Walker RW, Lee L, Costa DC, Livingston G, Ince PG, Perry R, McKeith I, Katona CL: Dementia with Lewy bodies: a comparison of clinical diagnosis, FP-CIT single photon emission computed tomography imaging and autopsy. J Neurol Neurosurg Psychiatry 2007;78:1176–1181.
29 Walker Z, Costa DC, Janssen AG, Walker RW, Livingstone G, Katona CL: Dementia with Lewy bodies: a study of post-synaptic dopaminergic receptors with iodine-123 iodobenzamide single-photon emission tomography. Eur J Nucl Med 1997;24: 609–614.
30 McKeith IG, Dickson DW, Lowe J, et al: Diagnosis and management of dementia with Lewy bodies: third report of the DLB consortium. Neurology 2005;65:1863–1872.
31 McKeith IG, Ballard CG, Harrison RW: Neuroleptic sensitivity to risperidone in Lewy body dementia. Lancet 1995;346:699.
32 Cummings JL, Street J, Masterman D, Clark WS: Efficacy of olanzapine in the treatment of psychosis in dementia with Lewy bodies. Dement Geriatr Cogn Disord 2002;13:67–73.
33 Takahashi H, Yoshida K, Sugita T, Higuchi H, Shimizu T: Quetiapine treatment of psychotic symptoms and aggressive behavior in patients with dementia with Lewy bodies: a case series. Prog Neuropsychopharmacol Biol Psychiatry 2003;27: 549–553.
34 Kurlan R, Cummings J, Raman R, Thal L: Quetiapine for agitation or psychosis in patients with dementia and parkinsonism. Neurology 2007;68:1356–1363.
35 Tiraboschi P, Hansen LA, Alford M, Merdes A, Masliah E, Thal LJ, Corey-Bloom J: Early and widespread cholinergic losses differentiate dementia with Lewy bodies from Alzheimer disease. Arch Gen Psychiatry 2002;59:946–951.
36 Beversdorf DQ, Warner JL, Davis RA, Sharma UK, Nagaraja HN, Scharre DW: Donepezil in the treatment of dementia with Lewy bodies. Am J Geriatr Psychiatry 2004;12:542–544.
37 Edwards KR, Hershey L, Wray L, Bednarczyk EM, Lichter D, Farlow M, Johnson S: Efficacy and safety of galantamine in patients with dementia with Lewy bodies: a 12-week interim analysis. Dement Geriatr Cogn Disord 2004;(suppl 1):40–48.
38 McKeith IG, Grace JB, Walker Z, Byrne EJ, Wilkinson D, Stevens T, Perry EK: Rivastigmine in the treatment of dementia with Lewy bodies: preliminary findings from an open trial. Int J Geriatr Psychiatry 2000;15:387–392.

Prof. Gabriel Gold
Department of Geriatrics and Rehabilitation, Hôpital des Trois-Chênes
3, chemin du Pont-Bochet
CH–1226 Thônex, Geneva (Switzerland)
Tel. +41 22 305 6530, Fax +41 22 305 6528, E-Mail gabriel.gold@hcuge.ch

Giannakopoulos P, Hof PR (eds): Dementia in Clinical Practice.
Front Neurol Neurosci. Basel, Karger, 2009, vol 24, pp 114–125

Significance of Brain Lesions in Parkinson Disease Dementia and Lewy Body Dementia

Kurt A. Jellinger

Institute of Clinical Neurobiology, Vienna, Austria

Abstract

Dementia is increasingly recognized as a common feature in patients with Parkinson disease (PD) and dementia with Lewy bodies (DLB), both sharing many clinical and morphological features and believed to form a continuum within the spectrum of Lewy body diseases. Based on a large autopsy series of parkinsonism (31–37% with dementia) and review of the recent literature, the pathological changes underlying cognitive impairment in PD with dementia (PDD) and DLB are discussed. PD cases with Lewy body stages 3–5, i.e. only mild to moderate cortical α-synuclein (αSyn) depositions, and no additional pathologies, are rarely associated with cognitive impairment, which is frequently seen in PD and DLB cases with considerable cortical and limbic αSyn load (increasing Lewy body densities) and/or associated widespread Alzheimer-type pathology. Clinicopathological studies show a negative relation between cognitive impairment and both cortical Lewy body pathology and Alzheimer type changes, suggesting that these either alone or in combination are major causes of cognitive dysfunction, while others related them to presynaptic αSyn aggregates. The neuropathology of PDD and DLB is similar, without significant differences between cortical and subcortical Lewy bodies and the pattern of synuclein pathology in the brainstem, but there are topographic differences in nigral lesions, more frequent affection of the hippocampal CA 2/3 subareas and more severe diffuse amyloid plaque load in the striatum of DLB. In conclusion, the pathology underlying cognitive impairment in PDD and DLB is heterogeneous, but there are some differences in the topography and severity of lesions between both phenotypes that need further evaluation.

Dementia has been increasingly recognized to be a common feature in patients with Parkinson disease (PD), especially in old age, referred to as PD dementia (PDD), and in dementia with Lewy bodies (DLB), which are believed to form phenotypes of a disease spectrum, characterized pathologically by deposition of α-synuclein (αSyn) within nerve cells (Lewy bodies, LBs) and dystrophic (Lewy) neurites in the central and autonomic nervous system, and clinically by a variable admixture of cognitive, neuropsychiatric, extrapyramidal, and vegetative features [1–3]. Clinical and pathological diagnostic criteria for PDD and DLB have been published recently [3–5], as well as interrater assessment results of αSyn pathology [6].

Dementia in PD with incidence rates of 95–112.5 per 1,000 patient-years (odds ratio for dementia in PD 3.5), a point prevalence close to 30% and a cumulative prevalence between 48 and 78% after 15 and 8 years' follow-up, respectively, is suggested to have a 4–6 times increased lifetime incidence rate compared to age-matched controls [5]. Prevalence estimates for DLB, depending on case criteria, range from 0 to 5% of the general population and from 0 to 30% of all dementia cases, with an incidence of 0.1 per year for the general population and 3.2 per year for new dementia cases [7]. A recent clinicopathological study confirmed essential clinical differences between PD with and without dementia and DLB: PDD patients were significantly older at death and had a shorter duration of illness and lower Mini-Mental State Examination (MMSE) scores than nondemented ones [8]. This chapter will review the morphological bases of cognitive impairment in PDD and DLB, their pathogenesis, mutual relationship and functional impact.

Morphological Substrates of Cognitive Impairment in Parkinson Disease

Brain lesions contributing to cognitive impairment in PD are heterogeneous, including dysfunction of subcortico-cortical networks due to neuron loss in brainstem and limbic areas, cholinergic deficit in cortical regions and thalamus, associated with neuron loss in the nucleus basalis of Meynert and decreased striatal dopaminergic function [9, 10], and widespread decrease in nicotinic acetylcholine receptors [11]. Frequent are limbic and cortical LBs and Alzheimer-type pathologies with loss of synapses and neurons [2], presynaptic αSyn aggregates [12], or variable combinations of these changes [2]. These changes may have common origins with mutual triggering due to synergistic reactions between αSyn, amyloid-β (Aβ) peptide and tau protein, the major protein markers of both PD and Alzheimer's disease (AD) that often may show morphological overlap with co-occurrence of lesions [8, 13–15].

In a 50-year autopsy series of 900 cases with clinical parkinsonism, pure LB disease was seen in 85%, but only 45% showed the morphological features of sporadic PD (brainstem predominant form or LB disease), 16% were associated with cerebrovascular lesions, 15% with Alzheimer-type pathology, 12.5% showing neuritic Braak stages 5 and 6; DLB was diagnosed in 9%, whereas 15% showed other degenerative disorders or secondary parkinsonism [16]. This differed from recent data of the UK Parkinson Brain Bank (63% PD, 29% other neurodegenerative disorders, 5% secondary parkinsonism and 3% others [14]).

Although a few cortical LBs are found in virtually all cases of sporadic PD, the impact of cortical LB and Alzheimer-type pathologies on cognitive impairment is a matter of discussion. Some studies have demonstrated that the number of LBs in the frontal cortex is the most significant predictor of cognitive status in PD [17] or that LB densities in the limbic cortex are a better predictor of dementia in PD than Alzheimer-type pathology [18–20]. Cognitive impairment is often correlated with the density of Lewy neurites and neuritic degeneration in the hippocampus and periamygdaloid cortex causing a disruption of the limbic loop and 'disconnection' from key areas similar to those described for the hippocampus in AD [21]. The density of both limbic LBs and neuritic plaques correlated well with dementia severity, suggesting that both lesions independently or synergistically contribute to dementia [22] or may have common origins with mutual triggering. Increasing cognitive decline (decreasing MMSE scores) with increasing pathological LB stages from 3 to 6, i.e. progression of αSyn pathology [23] was not confirmed by others [24–26]. PDD patients often have severe Alzheimer-type lesions [27] with or without neocortical atrophy [28], although quantitative stereological studies found no global loss of neocortical neurons, but could not exclude local neuron loss in specific subpopulations or in small but essential neocortical subregions in PD [29].

Although Alzheimer-type pathology is considered to represent a major cause of dementia in PD, it shows some differences. Comparative studies of neuritic AD stages and cognitive state assessed by MMSE in 55 cases of PD showed significant negative correlation between both parameters (fig. 1a). In contrast to severely demented 'pure' AD cases without parkinsonian signs of Braak stages 5 and 6 (fig. 1b), PDD and some DLB cases showed less frequent isocortical neuritic AD stages. There were no significant differences in the severity of neuritic AD lesions between PD and DLB cases with similar MMSE scores (fig. 1a). In PD, mild to moderate cognitive impairment (MMSE 15–24) was associated with Braak stages 2–4, while in aged parkinsonian subjects, the severity of neuritic AD lesions ranged from Braak stages 2 to 5 (fig. 1b). Since some PD brains showed cortical and/or limbic LBs, their synergistic effect in cognitive impairment can be assumed, but needs to be confirmed by future prospective clinicopathological studies.

In an autopsy series of 330 elderly patients with clinical parkinsonism (37.6% with dementia), only 3.2% of the demented subjects (MMSE <20) showed LB Braak stages 3–5, which was present in the majority of nondemented patients, while 37% of PDD cases revealed LB stages 4 or 5 with additional severe Alzheimer-type pathology (neuritic Braak stages 5 and 6) [16]. More than half of them showed strong relationship between the severity of αSyn and tau pathologies, particularly in the limbic system. DLB with low or high-grade Alzheimer-type lesions were seen in 32% of PPD patients, but 35% of diffuse DLB cases with mild AD lesions (amyloid plaques or tau pathology restricted to the limbic system, i.e., Braak stages lower than 4) did not show considerable cognitive dysfunction. Other degenerative parkinsonian disorders with superimposed Alzheimer-type pathology accounted for 7%, and AD, mixed-type dementia (AD + vascular encephalopathy) and subcortical vascular encephalopathy for 17%, while mild cerebrovascular lesions (lacunar state, few microinfarcts) were almost never associated with PDD (table 1). Neuropathology revealed lower brain

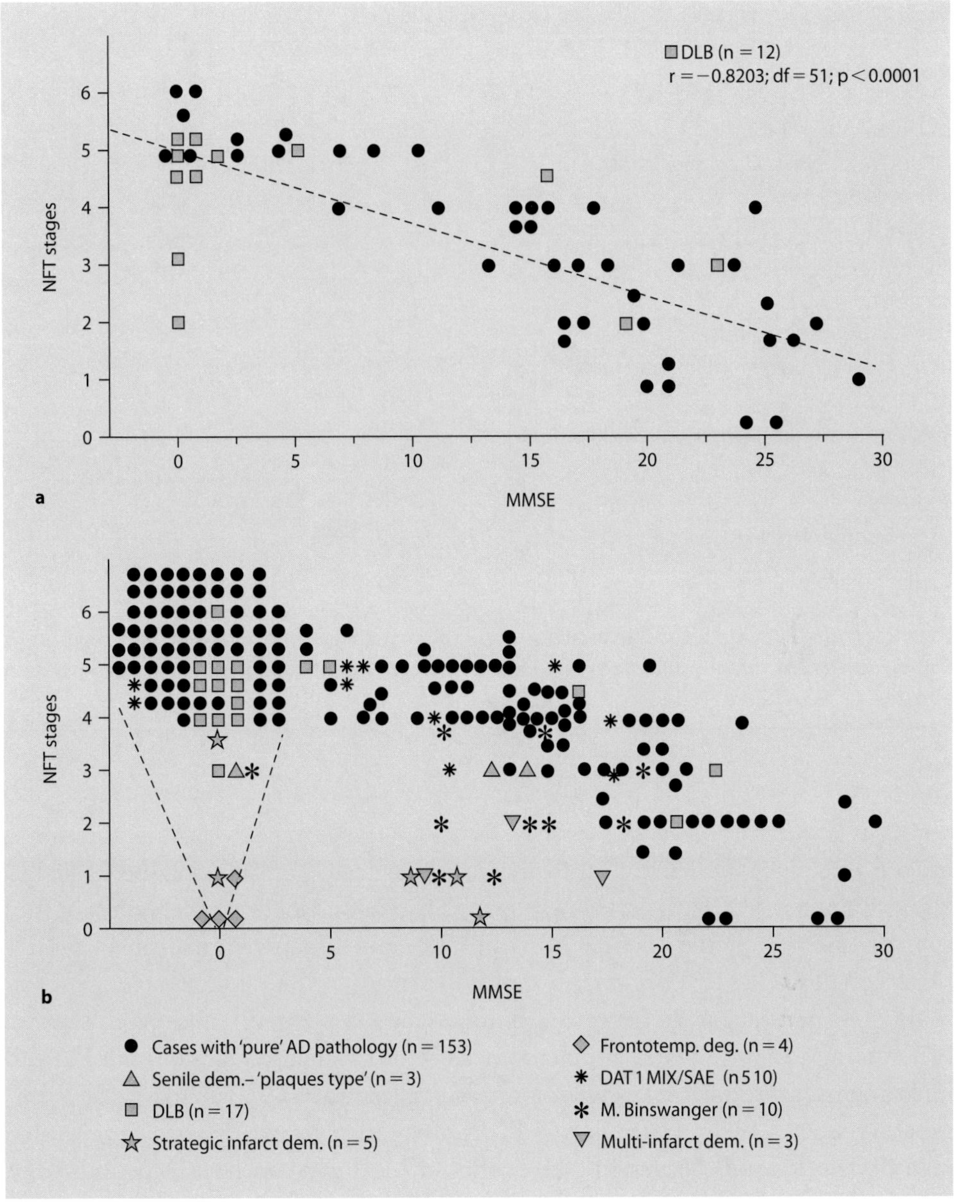

Fig. 1. Correlation between cognitive state (MMSE) and neuritic AD stages (NFT stages) in 55 autopsy cases of parkinsonism (**a**) and 205 aged subjects without parkinsonism (**b**).

weight in PDD than in nondemented PD and DLB, and significantly more severe Alzheimer-type lesions (neuritic Braak stages, cortical amyloid plaque load and generalized cerebral amyloid angiopathy, CAA) in PDD and DLB than in nondemented PD cases, while the morphological LB scores were only moderately increased in PDD (mean 4.5 vs. 4.1) and, in accordance with current diagnostic criteria, highest

Table 1. Pathology of parkinsonism with dementia (1988–2007)

Neuropathology	n	%
IPD (Braak stage 3–5)	5	3.2
IPD + CVLs (lacunar state, small infarcts)	1	0.6
IPD + AD (B/B 5–6)	57	37.0
IPD + VaE	7	4.5
IPD + MIX (AD + VaE)	4	2.6
LB variant of AD	18	11.7
Dementia with LBs, diffuse	30	19.5
IPD + other pathologies (hydrocephalus)	2	1.3
AD/MIX (AD + VaE)	17	11.0
Subcortical arteriosclerotic encephalopathy	2	1.3
PSP (+ AD), CBD	4	2.6
MSA + AD	5	3.2
Other disorders (Pick disease)	2	1.3
Total	154	100.0

IPD = Idiopathic PD; CVLs = cerebrovascular lesions; VaE = vascular encephalopathy; LB = Lewy body; PSP = progressive supranuclear palsy; CBD = corticobasal degeneration; MSA = multiple system atrophy.

in DLB (mean 5.5) [8]. Significantly increased cortical Aβ plaque load in PDD and DLB is in agreement with previous studies [23, 27, 30], whereas others did not find any correlation between cortical Aβ deposition and cognitive impairment in DLB [31]. Recent [^{11}C]-PIB PET studies showed cortical amyloid comparable to AD in some PDD patients, while fluorescence microscopy in postmortem sections showed PIB binding to Lewy bodies and neuromelanin in substantia nigra of both PD and PDD brainstem sections, not seen in controls, suggesting that PIB uptake in the brainstem may reflect PDD-related amyloid [32]. Two other recent PET studies revealed increased cortical Aβ burden in DLB similar to AD, but no increased cortical Aβ in PDD, PD without dementia and normal controls. These findings suggest that high cortical Aβ burden in DLB contributes to cognitive impairment in this disorder [32a, 32b]. In addition, striatal PIB retention in DLB, less in PDD, were related to less impaired motor functions [32b]. Increased amyloid load in meningeal and cortical vessels (CAA) in both PDD and DLB is also in agreement with previous studies [33]. In general, significant association between cognitive impairment and moderate association between morphological LB scores and cortical amyloid load, CAA, and neuritic Braak stage, the latter increasing with age, suggest an influence of AD-related pathology on the progression of the neurodegenerative process and, in particular, on cognitive decline in LB diseases. On the other hand, these factors in PD and DLB

Table 2. Major clinical and Alzheimer-related changes in Lewy body-related disorders, AD, and age-matched controls

	AD (n=30)	LBV/AD (n=26)	DDLB (n=31)	PDD (+AD) (n=11)	PD non-dem. (n=13)	Controls (n=7)	p
Age, years	79.0±5.3	79.8±4.9	76.0±6.1	77.1±5.1	74.3±5.4	77.7±3.2	
Male/female	25/5	8/18	9/22	3/8	5/8	5/2	
Duration, years	6.8±3.1*	5.9±2.3*	7.4±2.5#	7.3±3.2#	9.5±4.2*	–	*p < 0.01 vs. each other, #p < 0.05 vs. PD non-dem.
MMSE (n = 12/8)	0.5±0*	2.0±1.0*	15.1±5.2*	4.9±3.2*	24.7±1.0*	28.0±0.5	*p < 0.001vs. each other
Brain weight, g	1.081±48	1.182±112	1.206±92	1.188±86	1.246±51	1.337±118	
CERAD							
0	0	0	19	1	11	7	
A	0	0	9	3	1	0	
B	1	11	3	3	1	0	
C	29	15	0	4	0	0	
Braak stage	5.5±0.2*	4.76±0.2*	2.61±0.3	4.1±0.5*	2.1±0.3	1.3±0.2	*p < 0.01 vs. DDLB and PD non-dem.

DDLB = Diffuse DLB.

appear to be largely independent of coexisting vascular pathology, except in cases with severe cerebrovascular lesions or those related to neuritic AD pathology [8].

A comparison of major clinical/cognitive and AD-related morphological changes in 117 autopsy cases of LB-related disorders, AD (without other pathologies), and age-matched controls (table 2) showed longest disease duration in nondemented PD patients, lowest final MMSE scores in AD and DLB associated with AD (LBV/AD) and PDD. Brain weight in nondemented PD cases and controls was significantly higher than in all demented groups, and the neuritic Braak stages (highest in AD and LBV/AD followed by PDD) correlated well with the level of cognitive impairment and with progressive hippocampal atrophy in PD>PDD>AD [34] and the severity of involvement of the cholinergic system with more severe neuronal loss in nucleus basalis of Meynert in LBV/AD than in pure AD and non-demented PD [16], and widespread cholinergic cortical losses differentiating DLB and LBV/AD from classical AD [35, 36].

Neuropathological Comparison between Parkinson Disease Dementia and Dementia with Lewy Bodies

The hallmark of DLB is α-synucleinopathy manifested as LBs of the classical and cortical types and neuritic degeneration. LBs are scored semiquantiatively according to the severity and anatomical distribution, distinguishing a brainstem predominant (PD), limbic (or transitional) with predominant involvement of the limbic lobe and neocortical type with widespread cortical LBs [3, 37], but there is no accepted 'gold standard' for the pathological diagnosis of DLB as has been proposed for AD.

The neuropathology of PDD and DLB shows similarities and slight differences. The morphology and immunohistochemistry of cortical and subcortical LBs and the ascending spreading pattern of αSyn pathology with onset in the lower brainstem and progression via midbrain, dorsal forebrain, amygdala, limbic system, limbic mesocortex to the neocortex [38] do not significantly differ between both phenotypes, the late stages 5 and 6 of LB pathology (involvement of sensory association and prefrontal primary sensory and motor areas), suggesting transition between PD and DLB [2]. However, there are some deviations in the severity and distribution pattern of lesions in the substantia nigra compacta (more severe and predominant cell loss in the medioventral parts in PD/PDD vs. more severe damage to the dorsolateral parts in DLB), more frequent involvement by αSyn deposits of the neocortex and limbic system, in particular of the CA 2/3 subareas of hippocampus in DLB (79 vs. 36%). A major morphological difference is the significantly more frequent and more severe load with diffuse amyloid plaques and less severe tau pathology in the striatum in DLB, irrespective of the severity of cortical Alzheimer-type lesions, while nondemented PD cases are virtually free of striatal amyloid plaques [39, 40]. The globus pallidus is free of amyloid plaques, while few αSyn deposits were seen in 76% of DLB and in around 30% of PDD brains, but only in 10% of nondemented PD cases. Tau pathology in the striatum was also more frequent in DLB than in both PD and PDD, the incidence of negative cases being 70 vs. 82 and 100%, respectively (fig. 2). These findings support a morphological distinction between DLB and PDD, but also between PDD and nondemented PD, which, however, does not appear to be restricted to diffuse Aβ deposition in the striatum; the neuritic Alzheimer-type pathology is usually much more severe in both DLB and PDD.

The question whether PD, DPP and DLB are different entities or represent a single entity with distinct clinical and pathological phenotypes is still considered controversial. Some genetic and biochemical differences argue for a separation between DLB/PDD and AD [16], although neuritic Alzheimer-like lesions are frequently seen as a burden which is equivalent to that in AD and would fit to the diagnosis of definite AD according to the CERAD protocol. This particular type has been referred to as LB variant of AD (LBV/AD) [41, 42], while those with more prominent Alzheimer-type pathology and αSyn deposits mainly restricted to the amygdala have been considered a distinct form of α-synucleinopathy [43].

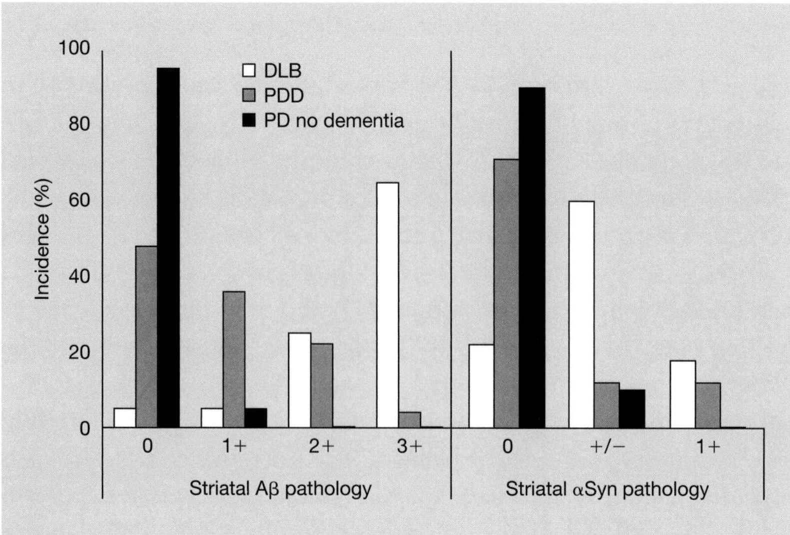

Fig. 2. Severity of Aβ and αSyn pathology in striatum in DLB, PDD and PD without dementia.

In a group of 57 prospectively assessed patients confirmed at autopsy (29 DLB, 28 PDD), an association between long duration of parkinsonism prior to dementia and less severe cortical αSyn pathology, lower CERAD plaque scores, but not neuritic Braak staging and more pronounced cortical cholinergic deficits were observed, not supporting the hitherto applied arbitrary clinical cut-off between PDD and DLB [44].

A study of 88 autopsy-proven cases of DLB showed much higher diagnostic accuracy in subjects with low Braak stages, but only 15% in those with severe AD pathology [25]. In a personal study of 103 cases of autopsy-proven DLB, the mean age at onset (parkinsonism 61%, dementia 31%) was 68 ± 12.7 SD years, mean survival from symptom onset 6.7 (range 1–16) years; patients with initial parkinsonism were younger than those with initial dementia (mean 63 vs. 70 years, $p = 0.002$). 62% showed low AD Braak stages (mean 3.5, mean age at death 75 years), 68% limbic/transitional (LB stages 5), and 22% diffuse cortical DLB (LB stage 6), 38% had high AD Braak stages (mean 4.6). Initial dementia, fluctuating cognition, and hallucinations strongly predicted shorter survival than initial parkinsonian symptoms and longer delay of dementia development (mean 5.6 vs. 3.3 years, $p < 0.001$). Sensitivity, specificity and positive predictive value of the McKeith criteria or probable AD were 0.60, 0.85, and 0.60, respectively. Clinical accuracy for DLB with low AD Braak stages was significantly higher than for patients with high Braak stages (70 vs. 22%) [26]. These two studies suggest that in DLB AD pathology has more influence on both the phenotype and diagnostic accuracy than cortical LB distribution.

Conclusions

The presence of αSyn-positive lesions in 7–71% of sporadic and familial AD even in the absence of subcortical LBs and the involvement of other brain areas, the colocalization of tau and αSyn epitopes in LBs as well as clinical and biochemical overlap between PD, PDD, DLB and AD with and without amygdala LBs suggest that the process of LB formation is triggered, at least in part, by AD pathology [2, 16]. This collision of two processes may occur in the same brain region or even within single cells in the human brain, e.g. in LRRK2 mutations [45] and in tg mice, induction of hyperphosphorylation of tau by αSyn in the MPTP model of parkinsonism [46], the association of phospho-tau and αSyn in both NFTs and LBs [47], and the in vitro promotion of tau aggregation by αSyn and vice versa [48], highlight the interface between these two and other misfolded proteins [49]. Others have suggested that amyloid rather than tau enhances αSyn pathology in human brain and tg mice [50]; interactions between αSyn, Aβ and tau may be molecular mechanisms in overlapping pathology of AD and PD/DLB [15, 51, 52]. However, it is unclear, whether there is a common underlying pathogenic mechanism inducing both neurodegenerative and fibrillary protein aggregates that are typical for different disease processes (double or triple amyloidosis) or if they represent a common final pathology leading to neuronal degeneration causing both movement and cognitive disorders. These and other recent data emphasize the necessity of proper neuropathological methods, in particular of specific immunohistochemistry for the different misfolded proteins as disease markers in the diagnostic evaluation of parkinsonian syndromes with and without cognitive impairment.

In conclusion, the pathogenesis, mutual relationship and functional impact of morphological lesions contributing to movement disorders and cognitive dysfunction/dementia in PD and DLB await further elucidation, in order to get better insights into the molecular disease mechanisms as a basis for better therapies.

References

1 Braak H, Sastre M, Bohl JR, de Vos RA, Del Tredici K: Parkinson's disease: lesions in dorsal horn layer I, involvement of parasympathetic and sympathetic pre- and postganglionic neurons. Acta Neuropathol 2007;113:421–429.

2 Jellinger KA: Morphological substrates of Parkinsonism with and without dementia. A retrospective clinico-pathological study. J Neural Transm 2007;(suppl 72):91–104.

3 McKeith IG, Dickson DW, Lowe J, et al: Diagnosis and management of dementia with Lewy bodies: third report of the DLB Consortium. Neurology 2005;65:1863–1872.

4 Dubois B, Burn D, Goetz C, Aarsland D, Brown RG, Broe GA, Dickson D, Duyckaerts C, Cummings J, Gauthier S, Korczyn A, Lees A, Levy R, Litvan I, Mizuno Y, McKeith IG, Olanow CW, Poewe W, Sampaio C, Tolosa E, Emre M: Diagnostic procedures for Parkinson's disease dementia: recommendations from the movement disorder society task force. Mov Disord 2007;22:2314–2324.

5 Emre M, Aarsland D, Brown R, Burn DJ, Duyckaerts C, Mizuno Y, Broe GA, Cummings J, Dickson DW, Gauthier S, Goldman J, Goetz C, Korczyn A, Lees A, Levy R, Litvan I, McKeith I, Olanow W, Poewe W, Quinn N, Sampaio C, Tolosa E, Dubois B: Clinical diagnostic criteria for dementia associated with Parkinson's disease. Mov Disord 2007;22:1689–1707
6 Alafuzoff I, Parkkinen L, Al-Sarraj S, et al: Assessment of α-synuclein pathology: a study of the BrainNet Europe Consortium. J Neuropathol Exp Neurol 2008;67:125–143.
7 Zaccai J, McCracken C, Brayne C: A systematic review of prevalence and incidence studies of dementia with Lewy bodies. Age Ageing 2005;34: 561–566.
8 Jellinger KA, Attems J: Prevalence and impact of vascular and Alzheimer pathologies in Lewy body disease. Acta Neuropathol 2008;115:427–436.
9 Caballol N, Marti MJ, Tolosa E: Cognitive dysfunction and dementia in Parkinson disease. Mov Disord 2007;(suppl 17):S358–S366.
10 Ziabreva I, Ballard CG, Aarsland D, Larsen JP, McKeith IG, Perry RH, Perry EK: Lewy body disease: thalamic cholinergic activity related to dementia and parkinsonism. Neurobiol Aging 2006;27: 433–438.
11 Fujita M, Ichise M, Zoghbi SS, Liow JS, Ghose S, Vines DC, Sangare J, Lu JQ, Cropley VL, Iida H, Kim KM, Cohen RM, Bara-Jimenez W, Ravina B, Innis RB: Widespread decrease of nicotinic acetylcholine receptors in Parkinson's disease. Ann Neurol 2006;59:174–177.
12 Kramer ML, Schulz-Schaeffer WJ: Presynaptic α-synuclein aggregates, not Lewy bodies, cause neurodegeneration in dementia with Lewy bodies. J Neurosci 2007;27:1405–1410.
13 Galpern WR, Lang AE: Interface between tauopathies and synucleinopathies: a tale of two proteins. Ann Neurol 2006;59:449–458.
14 Lashley T, Holton JL, Gray E, Kirkham K, O'Sullivan SS, Hilbig A, Wood NW, Lees AJ, Revesz T: Cortical α-synuclein load is associated with amyloid-β plaque burden in a subset of Parkinson's disease patients. Acta Neuropathol 2008;115:417–425.
15 Mandal PK, Pettegrew JW, Masliah E, Hamilton RL, Mandal R: Interaction between Aβ peptide and α synuclein: molecular mechanisms in overlapping pathology of Alzheimer's and Parkinson's in dementia with Lewy body disease. Neurochem Res 2006; 31:1153–1162.
16 Jellinger KA: Lewy body disorders; in Youdin MBH, Riederer P, Mandel SA, Battistin L, Lajtha A (eds): Degenerative Diseases of the Nervous System. New York, Springer Science, 2007, pp 267–343.
17 Mattila PM, Rinne JO, Helenius H, Dickson DW, Roytta M: α-Synuclein-immunoreactive cortical Lewy bodies are associated with cognitive impairment in Parkinson's disease. Acta Neuropathol 2000; 100:285–290.
18 Apaydin H, Ahlskog JE, Parisi JE, Boeve BF, Dickson DW: Parkinson disease neuropathology: later-developing dementia and loss of the levodopa response. Arch Neurol 2002;59:102–112.
19 Hurtig HI, Trojanowski JQ, Galvin J, Ewbank D, Schmidt ML, Lee VM, Clark CM, Glosser G, Stern MB, Gollomp SM, Arnold SE: α-Synuclein cortical Lewy bodies correlate with dementia in Parkinson's disease. Neurology 2000;54:1916–1921.
20 Kövari E, Gold G, Herrmann FR, Canuto A, Hof PR, Bouras C, Giannakopoulos P: Lewy body densities in the entorhinal and anterior cingulate cortex predict cognitive deficits in Parkinson's disease. Acta Neuropathol (Berl) 2003;106:83–88.
21 Mattila PM, Rinne JO, Helenius H, Roytta M: Neuritic degeneration in the hippocampus and amygdala in Parkinson's disease in relation to Alzheimer pathology. Acta Neuropathol (Berl) 1999; 98:157–164.
22 Harding AJ, Halliday GM: Cortical Lewy body pathology in the diagnosis of dementia. Acta Neuropathol 2001;102:355–363.
23 Braak H, Rub U, Jansen Steur EN, Del Tredici K, de Vos RA: Cognitive status correlates with neuropathologic stage in Parkinson disease. Neurology 2005;64:1404–1410.
24 Colosimo C, Hughes AJ, Kilford L, Lees AJ: Lewy body cortical involvement may not always predict dementia in Parkinson's disease. J Neurol Neurosurg Psychiatry 2003;74:852–856.
25 Weisman D, Cho M, Taylor C, Adame A, Thal LJ, Hansen LA: In dementia with Lewy bodies, Braak stage determines phenotype, not Lewy body distribution. Neurology 2007;69:356–359.
26 Jellinger KA: Re: in dementia with Lewy bodies, Braak stage determines phenotype, not Lewy body distribution. Neurology 2008;70:407–408.
27 Deramecourt V, Bombois S, Maurage CA, Ghestem A, Drobecq H, Vanmechelen E, Lebert F, Pasquier F, Delacourte A: Biochemical staging of synucleinopathy and amyloid deposition in dementia with Lewy bodies. J Neuropathol Exp Neurol 2006;65:278–288.
28 Ramirez-Ruiz B, Marti MJ, Tolosa E, Bartres-Faz D, Summerfield C, Salgado-Pineda P, Gomez-Anson B, Junque C: Longitudinal evaluation of cerebral morphological changes in Parkinson's disease with and without dementia. J Neurol 2005;252:1345–1352.

29 Pedersen KM, Marner L, Pakkenberg H, Pakkenberg B: No global loss of neocortical neurons in parkinson's disease: a quantitative stereological study. Mov Disord 2005;20:164–171.
30 Mastaglia FL, Johnsen RD, Byrnes ML, Kakulas BA: Prevalence of amyloid-β deposition in the cerebral cortex in Parkinson's disease. Mov Disord 2003;18: 81–86.
31 Thomas A, Ballard C, Kenny RA, O'Brien J, Oakley A, Kalaria R: Correlation of entorhinal amyloid with memory in Alzheimer's and vascular but not Lewy body dementia. Dement Geriatr Cogn Disord 2005; 19:57–60.
32 Maetzler W, Reimold M, Liepelt I, Solbach C, Leyhe T, Schweitzer K, Eschweiler GW, Mittelbronn M, Gaenslen A, Uebele M, Reischl G, Gasser T, Machulla HJ, Bares R, Berg D: [11C]PIB binding in Parkinson's disease dementia. Neuroimage 2008;39: 1027–1033.
32a Edison P, Rowe CC, Rinne JO, Ng S, Ahmed I, Kemppainen N, Villemagne VL, O'Keefe G, Nagren K, Chaudhuri R, Masters CL, Brooks DJ: Amyloid load in Parkinson's disease dementia and Lewy body dementia measured with [11C]PIB-PET. J Neurol Neurosurg Psychiatry 2008; in press.
32b Gomperts SN, Rentz DM, Moran E, Becker JA, Locascio JJ, Klunk WE, Mathis CA, Elmaleh DR, Shoup T, Fischman AJ, Hyman BT, Growdon JH, Johnson KA: Imaging amyloid deposition in Lewy body diseases. Neurology 2008;71:903–910.
33 Bertrand E, Lewandowska E, Pasennik E, Stepien T, Szpak GM, Dymecki J, Wierzba-Bobrowicz T: Cerebral amyloid angiopathy in idiopathic Parkinson's disease. Acta Neuropathol 2007;114: 308.
34 Burton EJ, McKeith IG, Burn DJ, O'Brien JT: Brain atrophy rates in Parkinson's disease with and without dementia using serial magnetic resonance imaging. Mov Disord 2005;20:1571–1576.
35 Camicioli R, Moore MM, Kinney A, Corbridge E, Glassberg K, Kaye JA: Parkinson's disease is associated with hippocampal atrophy. Mov Disord 2003; 18:784–790.
36 Tam CW, Burton EJ, McKeith IG, Burn DJ, O'Brien JT: Temporal lobe atrophy on MRI in Parkinson disease with dementia: a comparison with Alzheimer disease and dementia with Lewy bodies. Neurology 2005;64:861–865.
37 Dickson DW: Neuropathology and pathogenesis of dementia with Lewy bodies; in O'Brien J, Ames D, McKeith I, Chiu E (eds): Dementia with Lewy Bodies and Parkinson's Disease Dementia. London, Taylor & Francis, 2006, pp 149–166.
38 Braak H, Del Tredici K, Rub U, de Vos RA, Jansen Steur EN, Braak E: Staging of brain pathology related to sporadic Parkinson's disease. Neurobiol Aging 2003;24:197–211.
39 Jellinger KA, Attems J: Does striatal pathology distinguish Parkinson disease with dementia and dementia with Lewy bodies? Acta Neuropathol 2006;112:253–260.
40 Kalaitzakis ME, Graeber MB, Gentleman SM, Pearce RK: Striatal β-amyloid deposition in Parkinson disease with dementia. J Neuropathol Exp Neurol 2008.
41 Hansen L, Salmon D, Galasko D, Masliah E, Katzman R, DeTeresa R, Thal L, Pay MM, Hofstetter R, Klauber M, et al: The Lewy body variant of Alzheimer's disease: a clinical and pathologic entity. Neurology 1990;40:1–8.
42 Perneczky R, Mosch D, Neumann M, Kretzschmar H, Muller U, Busch R, Forstl H, Kurz A: The Alzheimer variant of Lewy body disease: a pathologically confirmed case-control study. Dement Geriatr Cogn Disord 2005;20:89–94.
43 Uchikado H, Lin WL, DeLucia MW, Dickson DW: Alzheimer disease with amygdala Lewy bodies: a distinct form of α-synucleinopathy. J Neuropathol Exp Neurol 2006;65:685–697.
44 Ballard C, Ziabreva I, Perry R, Larsen JP, O'Brien J, McKeith I, Perry E, Aarsland D: Differences in neuropathologic characteristics across the Lewy body dementia spectrum. Neurology 2006;67:1931–1934.
45 Giasson BI, Covy JP, Bonini NM, Hurtig HI, Farrer MJ, Trojanowski JQ, Van Deerlin VM: Biochemical and pathological characterization of Lrrk2. Ann Neurol 2006;59:315–322.
46 Duka T, Rusnak M, Drolet RE, Duka V, Wersinger C, Goudreau JL, Sidhu A: α-Synuclein induces hyperphosphorylation of Tau in the MPTP model of parkinsonism. FASEB J 2006;20:2302–2312.
47 Shao CY, Crary JF, Rao C, Sacktor TC, Mirra SS: Atypical protein kinase C in neurodegenerative disease II: PKCiota/lambda in tauopathies and α-synucleinopathies. J Neuropathol Exp Neurol 2006;65: 327–335.
48 Giasson BI, Forman MS, Higuchi M, Golbe LI, Graves CL, Kotzbauer PT, Trojanowski JQ, Lee VM: Initiation and synergistic fibrillization of tau and α-synuclein. Science 2003;300:636–640.
49 Soto C, Estrada LD: Protein misfolding and neurodegeneration. Arch Neurol 2008;65:184–189.
50 Pletnikova O, West N, Lee MK, Rudow GL, Skolasky RL, Dawson TM, Marsh L, Troncoso JC: Aβ deposition is associated with enhanced cortical α-synuclein lesions in Lewy body diseases. Neurobiol Aging 2005;26:1183–1192.

51 Obi K, Aklyama H, Kondo H, Shimomura Y, Hasegawa M, Iwatsubo T, Mizuno Y, Mochizuki H: Relationship of phosphorylated α-synuclein and tau accumulation to Aβ deposition in the cerebral cortex of dementia with Lewy bodies. Exp Neurol 2008;210:409–420.

52 Peuralinna T, Oinas M, Polvikoski T, Paetau A, Sulkava R, Niinisto L, Kalimo H, Hernandez D, Hardy J, Singleton A, Tienari PJ, Myllykangas L: Neurofibrillary tau pathology modulated by genetic variation of α-synuclein. Ann Neurol 2008;64:348–352.

Kurt A. Jellinger, MD
Institute of Clinical Neurobiology
Kenyongasse 18
AT–1070 Vienna (Austria)
Tel./Fax +43 1 526 6534, E-Mail kurt.jellinger@univie.ac.at

Giannakopoulos P, Hof PR (eds): Dementia in Clinical Practice.
Front Neurol Neurosci. Basel, Karger, 2009, vol 24, pp 126–134

Delineating Dementia with Lewy Bodies: Can Magnetic Resonance Imaging Help?

Armin von Gunten[a] · Reto Meuli[b]

[a]Service de Psychiatrie de l'Age Avancé, Département de Psychiatrie, Centre Hospitalier Universitaire Vaudois and University of Lausanne, Prilly; [b]Département de Radiodiagnostic et Radiologie Interventionnelle, Centre Hospitalization Universitaire Vaudois and University of Lausanne, Lausanne, Suisse

Abstract

As future treatments increasingly target the protein chemistry underlying the different dementias, it becomes crucially important to distinguish between the dementias during life. Neither specific protein nor genetic markers are as yet available in clinical practice. However, neuroimaging is an obvious candidate technique that may yield enhanced diagnostic accuracy when applied to the dementias. The physiopathology and anatomopathology is complex in dementia with Lewy bodies (DLB). Besides the relative sparing of medial temporal lobe structures in DLB in comparison to Alzheimer's disease, no clear signature pattern of cerebral atrophy associated with DLB has been established so far. Among others, one reason may be the difficulty in visualizing the small brain nuclei that are differentially involved among the dementias. While we think that structural magnetic resonance imaging neuroimaging should be part of the diagnostic workup of most dementia syndromes due to its usefulness in the differential diagnosis, its contribution to a positive diagnosis of DLB is as yet limited. The development of different neuroimaging techniques may help distinguish reliably DLB from other neurodegenerative disorders. However, in order to become accepted as part of standard care, these techniques must still prove their effectiveness under routine conditions such as those encountered by the general practitioner.

Clinical estimates of the prevalence of dementia with Lewy bodies (DLB) have been shown to be 50% or less of rates reported in autopsy series [1]. This discrepancy suggests that DLB cases are often not diagnosed correctly during life, a problem that persists to some extent in spite of internationally defined and regularly updated clinical criteria for DLB [2]. The clinically most important entities to be distinguished from DLB apart from normal aging are Alzheimer's disease (AD) and dementia associated with Parkinson's disease (PDD), both neurodegenerative diseases, as well as vascular dementia (VD). However, telling DLB apart from AD may be difficult as AD pathology is often associated with DLB pathology in brain autopsy studies [3]. Whether or not DLB and PDD are merely two variants of the same disorder is still open to debate.

In addition, even the subcortical variants of VD show some clinical overlap with the neurodegenerative disorders.

As future treatments will target the protein chemistry underlying the different dementias, it becomes increasingly important to distinguish between them during life, in particular between the various neurodegenerative disorders [4]. However, both treatments targeting specifically neurodegeneration in DLB and specific protein and genetic markers are not yet available in clinical practice [1]. Other markers with high specificity and sensitivity in differentiating neurodegenerative disorders are therefore of importance. Neuroimaging is an obvious approach that may yield enhanced diagnostic accuracy when applied to the dementias.

Neuroimaging reflects anatomical and physiological brain changes related to specific disease processes. In DLB, Lewy bodies (LB) and neuronal loss are found in the substantia nigra and pigmented brainstem nuclei (locus coeruleus, nucleus basalis of Meynert), the thalamus, and the hypothalamus. LB density varies between cortical areas and between patients. Limbic regions including the anterior cingulate cortex, insula, the entorhinal cortex, as well as the temporal lobes including the amygdala are usually more severely affected than other areas. Clinical studies suggest that medial temporal lobe changes often resulting in episodic memory deficits are less pronounced in DLB than in AD, which is in keeping with neuropathological studies. Visuoconstructive and executive functions are worse in DLB than in AD, but these findings are less consistently corroborated by neuropathology. However, the role played by LB and their relationship to the clinical features typically observed in DLB remain somewhat unclear [1]. The general picture is further complicated as an important part of the clinical observations in DLB may be secondary to accompanying AD lesions rather than LB, especially in late-onset DLB [3]. Furthermore, neuron loss, spongiform changes, or neurotransmitter imbalance may add to the elusiveness of anatomoclinical correlations in DLB [5].

It may thus be concluded that the physiopathology and anatomopathology in DLB is complex. If anything, limbic neocortical structures may be more involved and medial temporal lobe structures less involved in pure cases of DLB in comparison to AD. However, although interindividual variability, both clinical and neuropathological, may cast doubt on the existence of consistent brain changes in DLB, caution is warranted. If a consistent pattern exists, appropriate structural imaging techniques should be able to detect it. In fact, brain imaging may even detect significant brain anomalies well ahead of clinical disease manifestations. Technology is meant to help the clinician increase diagnostic accuracy at the earliest disease stages. Magnetic resonance imaging (MRI) is currently both the most sophisticated structural brain imaging technique due to its high contrast and a widely available tool recommended by many experts as a nearly mandatory approach to diagnosing cognitive disorders (look out for active body implants as a relative contraindication for MRI). Furthermore, MRI can be employed to study brain perfusion and vascular response to neuronal activity (functional MRI, fMRI) without the use of radioactive isotopes.

Functional Magnetic Resonance Imaging

fMRI has shown both diffuse hypoperfusion and a more focal occipital decrease similar to positron-emission tomography or single photon emission computed tomography (SPECT) studies [6]. Reduction is most pronounced in the visual association cortex compared to that in AD patients and could distinguish DLB from AD with good sensitivity and specificity. Posterior hypofunctioning may relate to spongiform changes in the occipital white matter [5] and in part corroborate visuoperceptive deficits that are clinically paramount in DLB [3]. The above pattern was found when subjects were scanned during resting cognitive state, without performing any specific task when being scanned. The use of specific cognitive tasks may help distinguish between different dementias [7]. Emerging studies suggest that fMRI may become a useful technique to detect both performance-dependent and performance-independent differences between various dementing disorders.

Morphological Magnetic Resonance Imaging

Besides its use in diagnosing secondary dementias (i.e. dementias due to neoplasias, strokes, infections, etc.), MRI is increasingly used to detect specific patterns of subcortical and cortical atrophy that might differentiate the various neurodegenerative diseases. Both qualitative and quantitative techniques to assess atrophy exist. Quantitative approaches include voxel-based morphometry (VBM) that is operator-independent and thought to be more reliable than the more qualitative analyses usually performed. However, even VBM cannot distinguish between brain areas with similar imaging properties producing no or very low contrast as in the case of adjacent brain nuclei and, for the time being, its application is limited to research settings.

In DLB, a diffuse cortical atrophy said to be less pronounced than that of typical AD has been described [6]. Atrophy may be absent or be considered an uncharacteristic feature of DLB [8]. The degree of ventricular enlargement did not distinguish AD from DLB [8]. The medial temporal lobe structures, in particular the hippocampus, are less atrophic in DLB patients than in those with AD [3, 8–11]. A third of DLB patients had normal medial temporal atrophy scores that correlated with age, especially in the head of the hippocampus [9, 10]. The preservation of the medial temporal lobe structures in DLB relative to AD may be secondary to reduced AD pathology in DLB [11]. Similarly, the parahippocampal area is less atrophic in DLB than in AD [10]. Differences of segmental hippocampal volumes between subjects with DLB and AD were observed across the whole length of the hippocampus [10]. A VBM study showed bilateral temporal grey matter volume loss sparing the medial portions including the hippocampus and the amygdala in the middle stages of DLB compared to normal controls [12]. In addition, there was a loss of the asymmetry normally observed in healthy subjects, with the right hippocampus being larger than the left one [10]. Patients with VD had somewhat greater medial temporal atrophy than those with DLB [9]. Thus, medial temporal atrophy is not specific to AD and – although its absence may be suggestive of a diagnosis of DLB – its sensitivity is limited [9].

A study showed bilateral grey matter volume loss in specific frontal lobe (Brodmann's areas 6 and 47) and insular cortex areas in the middle stages of DLB [12]. No differences in frontal grey matter volume between DLB and AD were observed. A VBM study confirmed grey matter loss in the insular and prefrontal cortex bilaterally as well as in the left premotor area [13] but grey matter loss observed in the frontal lobes may reflect concomitant AD pathology [11].

The presence of visuoconstructive deficits in DLB patients may suggest occipital lobe atrophy. However, these deficits are usually complex and related to temporo-occipital changes, which is in keeping with the absence of occipital lobe atrophy in 23 DLB patients compared to both AD and normal subjects [14]. Whole volume measures as used in this study may, however, be less accurate than differential analyses of selective volumetric changes of either grey or white matter. Another study using VBM made up for this shortcoming and found no grey matter changes in the occipital lobes [12]. Grey matter loss was also observed in the parietal lobes although this may, again, reflect concomitant AD pathology [11].

DLB is a neuropsychiatric disease eventually accompanied by serious behavioral and psychological symptoms that may be associated not only with cortical lesions but also with alterations in subcortical structures related to the limbic system. Thus, some of the emotional and possibly olfactory disturbances seen in DLB could be related to a dysfunction of the basal forebrain and suggest more focused loss in this brain region [13, 15]. Grey matter volume of the amygdala and the thalamus was preserved in DLB relative to AD [12]. Indeed, unlike AD, marked atrophy of the thalamus has not yet been reported as a feature of DLB. Thickness measures of the substantia innominata, that contains the cholinergic nucleus basalis Meynert, revealed greater atrophy in the DLB group when compared with the AD group. This finding corroborates both neuropathological studies and a somewhat better clinical response to acetylcholinesterase inhibitors in patients suffering from DLB [16]. The finding of significantly more decreased grey matter in the substantia innominata in DLB as compared to AD is confirmed by another study comparing 72 pairs of age- and gender-matched DLB and AD patients using VBM [11]. Although substantia innominata wasting showed a trend towards greater involvement in AD than in DLB, a closer look revealed a discrete loss with regard to uninvolved adjacent areas in DLB as opposed to AD that affected more indiscriminantly surrounding areas. Furthermore, patients with DLB as a group had regional grey matter loss in the dorsal midbrain and the hypothalamus [11]. Grey matter volume loss was greater in DLB than in AD. These brain regions contain cholinergic systems and have been shown to be altered in neuropathological studies of DLB. Furthermore, these changes are reminiscent of the progression of LB pathology in Parkinson's disease (PD) and may be similar in DLB. Structural studies have limited resolution however, and it is difficult to visualize specific small brain nuclei. Thus, both the small size of cholinergic nuclei and their wide and diffuse projections prevent visualizing the cholinergic system using structural MRI [12].

The presence of periventricular, white matter hyperintensities (WMH) and basal ganglia hyperintensities on MRI do not seem to distinguish AD from DLB, but they are clearly more extensive in DLB than in normal controls except perhaps for the near ubiquitous presence of frontal caps [17]. In contrast, global WMH volume was not significantly greater in DLB patients than in normal controls, while AD patients had a significantly greater WMH load [18]. The lack of an association between DLB and basal ganglia hyperintensities beyond that seen in AD indicates that these lesions may not be contributive to the development of parkinsonism in DLB [17]. Similarly, decreased occipital hypofunctioning revealed by dynamic neuroimaging [6] is unlikely to be correlated with WMH. This decrease may relate to spongiform white matter changes and is in keeping with the absence of occipital lobe atrophy as mentioned earlier [5, 14].

This survey shows that most studies look for differences between DLB patients and either normal or AD subjects. Although this is appropriate due to the high prevalence rates of normal aging and AD, the clinical reality confronts the clinician with more complex issues in terms of differential diagnosis. VD and its neuroimaging overlap in the normal and demented elderly is paramount and has received little attention in comparison with DLB despite clinical overlap between DLB and VD. Although DLB may be the cognitive-onset variant and PDD the motor-onset variant of the same disease, one might still wonder whether or not MRI can distinguish between the two variants. Indeed, DLB patients have greater grey matter atrophy in some temporal, parietal, and occipital areas than patients with PDD [19]. However, this study must be considered preliminary and others did not find such differences [20, 21]. MRI changes of the substantia nigra in PD and PDD can be visualized (fig. 1).

However, in one large study, no volume loss in the region of the substantia nigra was found in DLB [11]. Thus, we might hypothesize that visualizing the substantia nigra may help distinguish PDD from DLB, but to our knowledge no study directly compares substantia nigra volumes between DLB and PDD.

Neuroimaging is of limited interest in the advanced stages of the dementias when the specific diagnostic issues are less at stake. To be useful, neuroimaging markers should help identify specific neurodegenerative disorders with both high specificity and sensitivity at early dementia stages. Thus, newer studies try to identify precursor stages of the dementias, such as mild cognitive impairment (MCI). While the amnestic form of MCI as a precursor stage of AD and its classical hippocampal atrophy on MRI bears the bulk of these studies, a few investigations have looked into neuroimaging characteristics of MCI type prodromal for other dementing illnesses. One small study including 8 patients with probable PD and possible DLB precursor stages found more entorhinal cortex and hippocampal atrophy than in normal controls; these neuroimaging findings were similar but less pronounced than in MCI prodromal for AD. Greater enlargement of the third ventricle in PD/DLB-MCI compared to vascular MCI

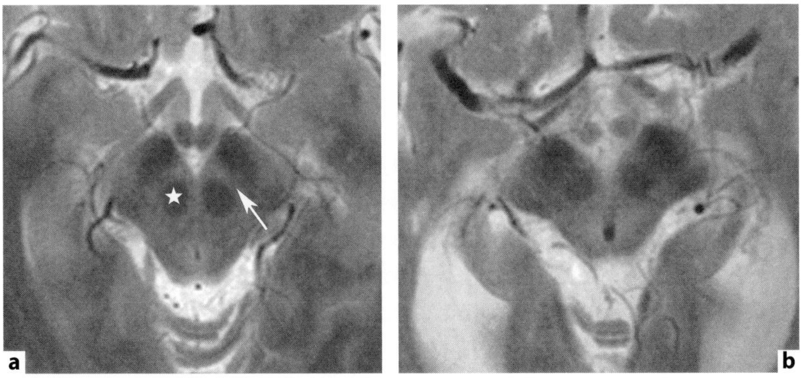

Fig. 1. Three Tesla T2-weighted magnetic resonance images in the axial plane at the level of the red nucleus (star) and substantia nigra (arrow on the pars compacta) in a normal subject (**a**) and in a PD patient with dementia (**b**) showing the global atrophy of the mesencephalon and the severe atrophy of the pars compacta of the substantia nigra.

was thought to reflect severe subcortical basal ganglion atrophy [22]. Furthermore, subjects with PD/DLB-MCI and concomitant vascular risk factors had more extensive subcortical white matter and basal ganglia lacunar infarcts and leucoaraiosis with greater bilateral frontal horn enlargement as opposed to those without vascular risk factors. This finding suggests that vascular lesions contribute to the development of cognitive impairment among PD/DLB-MCI subjects with vascular risk factors [22].

Cross-sectional diagnosis may be difficult in slowly progressing disorders such as DLB. Therefore, sequential assessments may be better suited to reach a definite diagnosis and sequential MRI scans may be helpful. A study with diagnostic post-mortem confirmation found that the progression of whole-brain atrophy and ventricular expansion in DLB was clearly lower, and in fact undistinguishable from normal controls, in comparison with AD, mixed AD/LB, frontotemporal lobe dementia with ubiquitin-only immunoreactive neuronal changes, progressive supranuclear paralysis, and corticobasal degeneration [4]. In DLB, the rate of whole-brain atrophy was only 0.4%/year, about a third of that of AD; the rate of ventricular expansion was 4.8%, about half that of AD. The mixed group of patients with AD and LB lesions had both rates of progression and memory deficits similar to those of subjects with pure AD. Another study was interested in the progression of WMH; progression was predicted by the baseline load of WMH, but their global volume increase was not significantly different between AD, PDD, and DLB [18].

Other Imaging Techniques

Although not the focus of this chapter, other brain imaging techniques are likely to play some role in the future. Visualization of pathological compounds using specific ligands is an expanding field in applied structural neuroimaging. As an example, beta amyloid burden as visualized using Pittsburgh Compound B-positron-emission tomography was lower and more variable in the precuneus and posterior cingulate in DLB patients than in those with AD [23]. Likewise, SPECT can be helpful in diagnosing DLB using dopamine transporter ligands such as ^{123}I-beta-CIT. Death of nigrostriatal dopaminergic neurons and decrease in presynaptic dopamine receptors can be demonstrated in DLB. Compared to PD without dementia, 12 h after withdrawal of antiparkinsonian therapy, these changes were more symmetrical in DLB despite the match for age and disease duration and did correlate with the severity of motor signs [24]. Diffusion tensor imaging allows for creating images of the diffusion of water in the brain and is a sensitive indicator of axonal changes. Using this technique, disruption of the white matter that connects posterior cingulate and lateral parietal regions was shown in DLB [25]. Similarly, a significant change in DLB was found in the precuneus, an area located in the medial parietal lobe that may be involved in visuospatial processing known to be altered in DLB and PD [26]. In AD subjects, diffusion-weighted changes were found in the left temporal lobe, which allowed to distinguish them from those in subjects with DLB. Imaging techniques tracing somatic changes secondary to neurodegenerative disorders are another evolving field. As an example, SPECT imaging of postganglionic sympathetic cardiac innervation using ^{123}I-metaiodobenzylguanidine has been shown to discriminate DLB from AD, with severe denervation being present in DLB [27].

Conclusions

Besides the relative sparing of medial temporal lobe structures in DLB in comparison with AD, no clear signature pattern of cerebral atrophy associated with DLB has been established so far [11]. This may be in part due to the variability in the definition of clinical cohorts and core clinical features as well as, of course, methodological issues regarding volumetric measures [11] such as the difficulty in visualizing small brain nuclei. As structural neuroimaging increases the in vivo diagnostic validity of neurodegenerative and VDs [28], it is now considered a nearly mandatory part in the diagnostic dementia workup. However, as few studies confront neuropathological and neuroimaging data, a diagnostic change due to neuroimaging may not always be justified as both vascular lesions and atrophic changes can be found in the elderly with no cognitive impairment.

While we think that structural MRI neuroimaging should be part of the diagnostic workup of most dementia syndromes due to its usefulness in the differential diagnosis, its contribution to a positive diagnosis of DLB is as yet limited. No optimized data exist and it is difficult to estimate the contribution of MRI to the diagnosis of patients in general practice. Nevertheless, some of the different neuroimaging techniques mentioned above may well be able to reliably distinguish DLB from other neurodegenerative disorders. However, in order to be accepted as part of the standard care, these techniques must still prove their effectiveness under routine conditions [28].

References

1 Geser F, Wenning GK, Poewe W, McKeith I: How to diagnose dementia with Lewy bodies: state of the art. Mov Dis 2005;20(suppl 12):S11–S20.

2 McKeith IG, Galasko G, Kosaka K, Perry EK, Dickson DW: Consensus guidelines for the clinical and pathologic diagnosis of dementia with Lewy bodies (DLB): a report of the consortium on DLB international workshop. Neurology 1996;47:1114–1124.

3 Salmon DP, Galasko D, Hansen LA: Dementia with Lewy bodies; in Hodes J (ed): Early-Onset Dementia: A Multidisciplinary Approach. Oxford, Oxford University Press, 2001, pp 305–318.

4 Whitwell JL, Jack CR, Parisi JE, Knopman DS, Boeve BF, Petersen RC, Ferman TJ, Dickson DW, Josephs KA: Rates of cerebral atrophy differ in different degenerative pathologies. Brain 2007;130: 1148–1158.

5 Higuchi M, Tashiro M, Arai H, Okamura N, Hara S, Higuchi S, Itoh M, Shin RW, Trojanowsky JQ, Sasaki H: Glucose hypometabolism and neuropathological correlates in brains of dementia with Lewy bodies. Exp Neurol 2000;162:247–256.

6 Ransmayr G, McKeith I: Demenzen mit Lewy-Körperchen und andere neurodegenerative Basalganglienerkrankungen; in Förstl H (ed): Lehrbuch der Gerontopsychiatrie und -psychotherapie, 2 Aufl. Stuttgart, Thieme, 2003.

7 Sauer J, Ffytche DH, Ballard C, Brown RG, Howard R: Differences between Alzheimer's disease and dementia with Lewy bodies: an fMRI study of task-related brain activity. Brain 2006;129:1780–1788.

8 Barber R, Ballard C, McKeith IG, Gholkar A, O'Brien JT: MRI volumetric study of dementia with Lewy bodies: a comparison with AD and vascular dementia. Neurology 2000;54:1304–1309.

9 Barber R, Gholkar A, Scheltens P, Ballard C, McKeith I, O'Brien J: Medial temporal lobe atrophy on MRI in dementia with Lewy bodies. Neurology 1999;52:1153–1158.

10 Barber R, McKeith IG, Ballard C, Gholkar A, O'Brien JT: A comparison of medial and lateral temporal lobe atrophy in dementia with Lewy bodies and Alzheimer's disease: magnetic resonance imaging volumetric study. Dement Geriatr Cogn Disord 2001;12:198–205.

11 Whitwell JL, Weigand SD, Shiumg MM, Boeve BF, Ferman TJ, Smith GE, Knopman DS, Petersen RC, Benarroch EE, Josephs KA, Jack CR Jr: Focal atrophy in dementia with Lewy bodies on MRI: a distinct pattern from Alzheimer's disease. Brain 2007; 130:708–719.

12 Burton EJ, Karas G; Paling SM, Barber R, Williams ED, Ballard CG, McKeith IG, Scheltens P, Barkhof F, O'Brien JT: Patterns of cerebral atrophy in dementia with Lewy bodies using voxel-based morphometry. Neuroimage 2002;17:618–630.

13 Brenneis C, Wenning GK, Egger KE, Schocke M, Trieb T, Seppi K, Marksteiner J, Ransmayr G, Benke T, Poewe W: Basal forebrain atrophy is a distinctive pattern in dementia with Lewy bodies. Neuroreport 2004;15:1711–1714.

14 Middelkoop HA, van der Flier WM, Burton EJ, Lloyd AJ, Paling S, Barber R, Ballard C, McKeith JG, O'Brien JT: Dementia with Lewy bodies and AD are not associated with occipital lobe atrophy on MRI. Neurology 2001;57:2117–2120.

15 Hanyu H, Tanaka Y, Shimizu S, Sakurai H, Iwamoto T, Abe K: Differences in MR features of the substantia innominata between dementia with Lewy bodies and Alzheimer's disese. J Neurol 2005;252:482–484.

16 Hanyu H, Shimizu S, Tanaka Y, Hirao K, Iwamoto T, Abe K: MR features of the substantia innominata and therapeutic implications in dementias. Neurobiol Aging 2007;28:548–554.

17 Barber R, Scheltens P, Gholkar A, Ballard C, McKeith I, Ince P, O'Brien J: White matter lesions on magnetic resonance imaging in dementia with Lewy bodies, Alzheimer's disease, vascular dementia, and normal aging. J Neurol Neurosurg Psychiatry 1999;67:66–72.

18 Burton EJ, McKeith IG, Burn DJ, Firbank MJ, O'Brien JT: Progression of white matter hyperintensities in Alzheimer disease, dementia with Lewy bodies, and Parkinson disease dementia: a comparison with normal aging. Am J Geriatr Psychiatry 2006;14:842–849.

19 Beyer MK, Janvin CC, Larsen JP, Aarsland D: A magnetic resonance imaging study of patients with Parkinson's disease with mild cognitive impairment and dementia using voxel-based morphometry. J Neurol Neurosurg Psychiatry 2007;78:254–259.

20 Burton EJ, McKeith IG, Burn DJ, Williams ED, O'Brien JT: Cerebral atrophy in Parkinson's disease with and without dementia: a comparison with Alzheimer's disease, dementia with Lewy bodies and controls. Brain 2004;127:791–800.

21 Seppi K, Rascol O: Dementia with Lewy bodies and Parkinson disease with dementia: can MRI make the difference? Neurology 2007;69:717–718.

22 Meyer JS, Huang J, Chowdhury MH: MRI confirms mild cognitive impairments prodromal for Alzheimer's, vascular, and Parkinson-Lewy body dementias. J Neurol Sci 2007;257:97–104.

23 Rowe CC, Ng S, Ackermann U, Gong SJ, Pike K, Savage G, Cowie TF, Dickinson KL, Maruff P, Darby D, Smith C, Wookward M, Merory J, Tochon-Danguy H, O'Keefe G, Klunk WE, Mathis CA, Price JS, Masters CL, Villemagne VL: Imaging beta-amyloid burden in aging and dementia. Neurology 2007; 68:1718–1725.

24 Ransmayr G, Seppi K, Donnemiller E, Luginger E, Marksteiner J, Riccabona G, Poewe W, Wenning GK: Striatal dopamine transporter function in dementia with Lewy bodies and Parkinson's disease. Eur J Nucl Med 2001;28:1523–1528.

25 Firbank MJ, Blamire AM, Krishnan MS, Teodorczuk A, English P, Gholkar A, Harrison RM, O'Brien JT: Atrophy is associated with posterior cingulate white matter disruption in dementia with Lewy bodies and Alzheimer's disease. Neuroimage 2007;36:1–7.

26 Firbank MJ, Blamire AM, Krishnan MS, Teodorczuk A, English P, Gholkar A, Harrison RM, O'Brien JT: Diffusion tensor imaging in dementia with Lewy bodies and Alzheimer's disease. Psychiat Res Neuroimaging 2007;155:135–145.

27 Yoshita M, Taki J, Yamada M: A clinical rele for ^{123}I-MIBG myocardial scintigraphy in the distinction between dementia of the Alzheimer's-type and dementia with Lewy bodies. J Neurol Neurosurg Psychiatry 2001;71:583–588.

28 Hentschel F, Kreis M, Damian M, Krumm B, Fröhlich L: The clinical utility of structural neuroimaging with MRI for diagnosis and differential diagnosis of dementia: a memory clinic study. Int J Geriatr Psychiatry 2005;20:645–650.

Dr. Armin von Gunten
Service de Psychiatrie de l'Age Avaucé (SUPAA)
Département de Psychiatrie, Centre Hospitalier Universitaire Vaudois and University of Lausanne
Route du Mont, CH–1008 Prilly (Switzerland)
Tel. +41 21 643 62 67, Fax +41 21 643 62 38, E-Mail armin.von-gunten@chuv.ch

Giannakopoulos P, Hof PR (eds): Dementia in Clinical Practice.
Front Neurol Neurosci. Basel, Karger, 2009, vol 24, pp 135–139

Pharmacotherapy of Parkinson Disease Dementia and Lewy Body Dementia

Serge Gauthier

McGill Center for Studies in Aging, Montréal, Que., Canada

Abstract

The pharmacotherapy of Parkinson disease dementia and Lewy body dementia with cholinesterase inhibitors and selected psychotropic drugs is relatively new. Review of literature supplemented by expert opinion. Cholinesterase inhibitors can be used by primary care practitioners and specialists, with often clinically meaningful results. Primary care practitioners play an essential role in the diagnosis and management of patients with these conditions.

Although in many countries the management of Parkinson disease dementia (PDD) and Lewy body dementia (DLB) is handled by specialists (predominantly neurologists), the primary care practitioner (PCP) plays an essential role in the care of patients with these conditions. The PCP is the one who detects in one of his patients an unusual presentation of dementia suggesting DLB (early and prominent visual hallucinations, fluctuations of alertness, spontaneous parkinsonism), or detects a decline in cognitive abilities in a patient who up to now has been stable with his Parkinson's disease (PD). The PCP can rule out delirium caused by infections, dehydration, metabolic factors, drug toxicity or a new neurological event. After the diagnosis of DLB or PDD has been made [see the chapter by Gold, pp. 107–113, for diagnostic criteria] by the PCP with or without confirmation by a specialist, pharmacotherapy can be initiated. The immediate improvement of symptoms in these conditions is often quite impressive and will provide satisfaction to the patient, his family and the treating physician. The randomized placebo-controlled evidence base for the medications used for these conditions is relatively limited compared to that of Alzheimer's disease (AD), but the clinical response is greater, at least in the short-term. This chapter will summarize the available literature and will provide practical advice in the use of currently available drugs for PDD and DLB. Although the pathological substrate of PDD and DLB is very similar [see the chapter by Jellinger, pp. 114–125], they have somewhat different

Table 1. Pharmacotherapy of PDD

Step 1	Step 2	Step 3
Phase out anticholinergic drugs, then amantadine, dopamine agonists, MAOB inhibitors	Decrease slowly levodopa and COMT inhibitors as low as tolerated, trying to preserve mobility and motor autonomy as much as possible	Start a ChEI (rivastigmine, donepezil, galantamine) and titrate up as tolerated If absolutely required: low doses of quetiapine, starting at 12.5 mg per day

pharmacotherapy. Thus the management of PDD will be discussed separately from DLB.

Pharmacotherapy of Parkinson Disease Dementia

PDD is diagnosed in the context of someone who has had classic PD motor symptoms for some time (resting tremor, bradykinesia, rigidity, often with some gait instability) and has been on related medications (anticholinergic drugs, amantadine, levodopa, dopamine agonists, COMT inhibitors, MAOB inhibitors). PDD symptoms such as visual hallucinations and fluctuations of alertness are first treated by withdrawing in sequence as much of the PD medication other than levodopa and COMT inhibitors as possible (table 1). If not successful, levodopa and COMT inhibitors may have to be lowered slowly, taking into account the control of motor symptoms. Patients are then started on a cholinesterase inhibitor (ChEI). The choice of ChEI is based on level of evidence and tolerability. Rivastigmine would be selected first by most clinicians [1], using the once a day transdermal patch if available rather than the oral twice a day tablet, with donepezil and galantamine as alternative. A low dose of an atypical antipsychotic may be required at any point if the neuropsychiatric symptoms (particularly delusions and agitation/agressivity) require immediate treatment: the best evidence is for clozapine [2] but clinically most clinicians will use quetiapine despite the lack of evidence from randomized clinical trials, principally because the doses can be increased progressively from 12.5 mg upwards without the need for hematologic monitoring [3, 4]. Although risperidone and olanzapine are atypical neuroleptics, they should not be used as they have been associated with clinically significant deterioration of the motor signs of parkinsonism in patients with PDD.

It should be noted that there are other neuropsychiatric complications of PD that require the attention of the PCP: depression, anxiety, psychosis, sleep disorders, gambling and other impulse control disorders [5]. The response to treatment can be assessed by the patient himself (which would be less common in AD) and his

Table 2. Pharmacotherapy of DLB

Step 1
Start a ChEI (rivastigmine, donepezil, galantamine) and titrate up as tolerated
For REM sleep disorder: clonazepam at bedtime
For associated motor features: try levodopa but stop if not effective or increasing hallucinations
Only if absolutely required: low doses of quetiapine, starting at 12.5 mg per day

entourage, who usually report a reduction of visual hallucinations and an increase in clarity of thinking within 2 months of starting a ChEI. The Mini-Mental State Examination [6] is often normal at the start of treatment since it is insensitive to the executive impairment associated with PDD and thus not very useful. Tests specific to executive function, attention or reaction time, and questionnaires for monitoring fluctuating attention have been tested in clinical trials [7]. The Montreal Cognitive Assessment is a promising test for daily clinical practice because it includes items relevant to executive functions and can be completed in less than 10 min [8].

The natural history of PDD once treatment has been initiated is stability of cognition for some months, until complications from the motor components of PD occur: falls and dysphagia leading to aspiration pneumonia. ChEI should be continued until the stage of severe dementia. There are insufficient data for or against recommending memantine in PDD.

Pharmacotherapy of Lewy Body Dementia

Most patients with DLB are not yet on medication when the diagnosis is made. The treating physician can thus start immediately with a ChEI (table 2). Based on evidence from randomized clinical trials, most clinicians will try rivastigmine first [9], with donepezil a close second, followed by galantamine. The efficacy is clinically as good as for PDD, and possibly more than in AD, considering the more severe cholinergic cortical deficits in PDD and DLB [10]. There is also the possibility that ChEI reduce cortical Aβ in the brain parenchyma [11]. The duration of benefit may be a little longer than in PDD because the motor complications of DLB occur later, but not as long as with AD. The safety of ChEI appears to be as good for DLB as it is for AD [12], although REM sleep disorder is more frequent, requiring clonazepam at bed time. On the other hand, these patients are more sensitive to drug withdrawals that patients with AD: a progressive withdrawal of ChEI may be required rather than abrupt cessation [13].

Neuroleptics (both typical and atypical) must be avoided because of the risk of neuroleptic hypersensitivity, which is associated with significant morbidity and mortality [14]. Nevertheless, atypical neuroleptics are sometimes required if all other treatments fail to control disturbing visual hallucinations, delusions and agitation. The least harmful appear to be quetiapine. A ChEI should always be tried first, unless there is a real urgency to control the behavioral symptoms.

Levodopa is often tried in DLB when motor symptoms become prominent, but the response to levodopa is not as prominent as in PD.

Conclusions

The management of PDD and DLB includes identification of problem symptoms, which will change over time, appropriate use of nonpharmacological interventions (education, coping strategies, targeted behavioral interventions), and judicious use of available medications [14, 15]. The positive results in PDD and DLB have opened the way for the treatment of other parkinsonian syndromes with ChEI [16]. The clinically meaningful responses to pharmacotherapy in PDD and LBD provide a great encouragement to patients, families and their treating physicians.

Acknowledgement

Special thanks to Dr. Michel Panisset for sharing his expertise in movement disorders over the years and for reviewing the manuscript.

References

1 Emre M, Aarsland D, Albanese A, Byrne EJ, Deuschl G, DeDyn PP, Durif F, Kulisevsky J, van Laar T, Lees A, Poewe W, Robillard A, Rosa MM, Wolters E, Quarg P, Tekin S, Lane R: Rivastigmine for dementia associated with Parkinson's disease. N Engl J Med 2004;351:2509–2518.

2 The Parkinson Study Group: Low-dose clozapine for the treatment of drug-induced psychosis in Parkinson's disease. N Engl J Med 1999;340:757–763.

3 Juncos JL, Roberts VJ, Evatt ML, Jewart RD, Wood CD, Potter LS, Jou HC, Yeung PP: Quatiapine improves psychotic symptoms and cognition in Parkinson's disease. Mov Disord 2004;19:29–35.

4 Prohorov T, Klein C, Miniovitz A, Dobronevsky E, Rabey JM: The effect of quetiapine in psychotic Parkinsonian patients with and without dementia. J Neurol 2006;253:171–175.

5 Ferreri F, Agbokou C, Gauthier S: Recognition and management of neuropsychiatric complications in Parkinson's disease. Can Med Assoc J 2006;175: 1545–1552.

6 Folstein MF, Folstein SE, McHugh PR: 'Mini-Mental State': a practical method for grading the cognitive state of patients for the clinician. J Psychiat Res 1975;12:189–198.

7 Camicioli R, Gauthier S: Clinical trials in Parkinson's dementia and dementia with Lewy bodies. Can J Neurol Sci 2007;34(suppl 1):S109–S117.

8 Nasreddine S, Phillips NA, Bedrrian V, et al: The Montreal Cognitive Assessment, MoCA: a brief screening tool for mild cognitive impairment. J Am Geriatr Soc 2005;53:695–699.

9 McKeith I, Del Ser T, Spano PF, Emre M, Wesnes K, Anand R, Cicin-Sain A, Ferrara R, Spiegel R: Efficacy of rivastigmine in dementia with Lewy bodies: a randomized, double-blind, placebo-controlled international study. Lancet 2000;356:2031–2036.

10 Bohnen NI, Kaufer DI, Ivanco LS, Lopresti B, Koepper RA, Davis JG, Mathis CA, Moore RY, DeKosky ST: Cortical cholinergic function is more severely affected in Parkinsonian dementia than in Alzheimer's disease. Arch Neurol 2003;60:1745–1748.
11 Ballard CG, Chalmers KA, Todd C, McKeith IG, O'Brien JT, Wilcock G, Love S, Perry EK: Cholinesterase inhibitors reduce cortical Aβ in dementia with Lewy bodies. Neurology 2007;68:1726–1729.
12 Ballard C, Lane R, Barone P, Ferrera R, Tekin S: Cardiac safety of rivastigmine in Lewy body and Pakinson's disease dementias. Int J Clin Pract 2006;60:639–645.
13 Pakrasi S, Thomas A, Mosimann UP, Cousins DA, Lett D, Burn DJ, O'Brien JT, McKeith IG: Cholinesterase inhibitors in advanced dementia with Lewy bodies: increase or stop? Int J Geriat Psychiatry 2006;21:719–721.
14 Barber R, Panikkar A, McKeith IG: Dementia with Lewy bodies: diagnosis and management. Int J Geriatr Psychiatry 2001;16:S12–S18.
15 Kaufer DI: Pharmacologic treatment expectations in the management of dementia with Lewy bodies. Dement Geriatr Cogn Disord 2004;17(suppl 1):32–39.
16 Liepelt I, Maetzler W, Blaicher HP, Gasser T, Berg D: Treatment of dementia in parkinsonian syndromes with cholinesterase inhibitors. Dement Geriat Cogn Disord 2007;23:251–267.

Serge Gauthier, MD, FRCPC
McGill Center for Studies in Aging
6825 LaSalle Blvd.
Montréal, QC, H4H 1R3 (Canada)
Tel. +1 514 766 1009, Fax +1 514 888 4050, E-Mail Serge.gauthier@mcgill.ca

Giannakopoulos P, Hof PR (eds): Dementia in Clinical Practice.
Front Neurol Neurosci. Basel, Karger, 2009, vol 24, pp 140–148

Clinical Features and Diagnosis of Frontotemporal Dementia

Andrew Kertesz

St. Joseph's Hospital, University of Western Ontario, London, Ont., Canada

Abstract

Frontotemporal degeneration (FTD), formerly known as Pick's disease has become recognized as a distinct and relatively common entity encompassing behavioural (bvFTD language (PPA) and extrapyramidal (CBD/PSP) presentations. Further clinical subdivisions such as semantic dementia (SD), and pathological subtypes such as mesial temporal sclerosis increase the complexity of diagnosis. The relatively younger age of onset, the typical presentations of syndromes and focal asymmetrical frontotemporal atrophy on imaging allows experienced clinicians to make the diagnosis confidently as long as the overlap between the syndromes is recognized. There is also an overlap with ALS pathologically and clinically. The underlying histology in FTD/Pick complex is ubiquitin positive tau and synuclein negative neuronal inclusions (FTLD-U) in more than half of autopsies and tau positive CBD/PSP/ Pick bodies (FTLD-T) in the rest. The clinical syndromes of bvFTD and SD are likely associated with FTLD-U and PPA/CBDS/PSP with FTLD-T, but there is too much overlap to predict the pathology from the clinical syndromes reliably. The ubiquitin-tau pathological dichotomy is best considered under the Pick complex umbrella to allow for the significant overlap. So far trazodone in behavior and galantamine in aphasia had symptomatic benefit in small trials and SSRI-s and antipsychotics in uncontrolled reports were used as symptomatic therapies. Recent discoveries of tau and progranulin (in the ubiquitin-positive cases) mutations on chromosome 17 and other mutations on chromosome 3 and 9 in the high incidence of autosomal dominant families and a common protein abnormality, the TDP-43 in FTLD-U and ALS are likely to be important in finding therapeutic targets.

Frontotemporal dementia (FTD) used to be called Pick's disease (PiD). Many would prefer to continue using the eponymic term because of its obvious symmetry to Alzheimer's disease (AD), for the sake of lay audiences and for historical accuracy; but pathologists restricted the use of the term for cases with Pick body histology. Pick's initial case of a progressive aphasic patient with behavioral disturbances had only anatomical examination without any microscopic data, but the clinical description and its relationship to focal atrophy is the basis of the syndrome

[1]. Frontotemporal atrophy was demonstrated with increasing frequency in vivo, first with CT then MRI and SPECT. However, instead of shifting the diagnosis of PiD back to the clinic, several studies applied new labels such as frontal lobe degeneration [2] or dementia of the frontal lobe type and subsequently frontotemporal dementia (FTD) [3] mainly for the behavioral presentation. The aphasic presentation was described again as a separate disease [4], but it became evident that they are closely related and that there is an extrapyramidal component as well, and the term Pick complex was suggested for the overall designation of all the clinical and pathological subtypes [5]. Frontotemporal lobar degeneration is also used, but inconsistently for the extrapyramidal components [6]. The terminological proliferation continues but a glossary at the end of the chapter may be helpful to navigate.

The Behavioral Variant

This is the commonest presentation with three major components often appearing together, but there exists some degree of separation of these by several years and a sequential accumulation of symptoms.

(1) The illness may begin with insidious changes, at times loss of executive function, apathy and disinterest which may be mistaken for depression. Initially, the inability to plan, or carry out complex tasks may be labeled a 'dysexecutive syndrome'. The patient is often inattentive, indecisive, impulsive and distractible. These symptoms are not very specific and occur in other conditions.

(2) The appearance of the symptoms of disinhibition is diagnostic but it may suggest a manic psychosis or an obsessive-compulsive or a sociopathic personality disorder [7]. Childish behavior, rudeness, inappropriate sexual remarks, impatient, careless driving, excessive spending or hoarding of certain items, inappropriate joking, perseverative routines, compulsive roaming, insistence of certain foods, excessive food intake, neglect of personal hygiene, disinterest in the immediate family, or others are the most characteristic features. The combination of hyperorality, hypersexuality and utilization behavior led to comparison with the 'Kluver-Bucy syndrome' [8].

(3) The personality change often prompts the family to say that the patient is not the same person any more. Pilfering, shoplifting, swearing, undressing in public, unexpected urinary frequency and fecal incontinence rapidly bring the patient to the physician, sometimes after the police is involved. When the striking disinhibition and asocial behavior appear in a middle-aged person between 40 and 65 years of age, the diagnosis should not be difficult, but FTD is often misdiagnosed under various psychiatric labels. Progressive language loss or aphasia (PA) is often superimposed or appears simultaneously and should be another diagnostic cue.

Primary Progressive Aphasia

Aphasia was described by Pick as part of circumscribed frontotemporal atrophy, but relabeled as primary progressive aphasia (PPA) later [4]. The relatively isolated language disturbance in the first 2 years of the illness was suggested as the operational definition of PPA. However, many cases have behavioral or extrapyramidal features which appear before 2 years. Variations of this terminology, particularly progressive nonfluent aphasia [9], and pure progressive aphemia [10] have been used. The condition was considered a separate entity for a while, but evidence was presented to consider it part of Pick complex/FTD [5]. The initial presentation of PPA is often with word finding difficulty, or anomia. In this respect, PPA patients are not much different from Alzheimer patients, except they have relatively preserved memory and non-verbal cognition. AD patients, on the other hand, by the time they show aphasic difficulty, usually have significant memory loss, disorientation, visuospatial and other cognitive impairment. The aphemic patients present with stuttering or slow, segmented speech and verbal apraxia, which includes articulatory difficulty and phonological paraphasias [10]. These patients are less likely to be mistaken for AD. A progressive limb apraxia can be a prominent feature indicating a clinical overlap between PPA and the apraxic-extrapyramidal syndrome of CBD.

A progressive loss of language output is called 'logopenia', defined as prominent word finding difficulty, but the phrase length is still longer than four words and syntax is preserved [11], and this is a common feature of PPA or secondary PA following the behavioral variant (bvFTD). Later, a logopenic variety was separated with different definition, such as prominent paraphasias and repetition disturbance, but many of these patients turn out to have AD. Comprehension, nonverbal intelligence and episodic memory are demonstrably maintained. Broca's aphasia with agrammatism is more characteristic of stroke patients, but it may be seen in PPA as a transient stage, usually progressing with increasing word finding difficulty to mutism. The course is variable, may be quite prolonged, but sometimes patients who develop pathology in the basal ganglia or motor neuron disease, progress quickly and develop difficulty with swallowing and choking [5]. Mutism has been considered characteristic of PiD, and it tends to be the end-stage of all forms of FTD, even those which start with behavioral abnormalities.

The differential diagnosis of PPA is most often AD, especially if memory complaints are present or vascular dementia, until the extrapyramidal or behavioral features make their appearance or the language deficit remains prominent and fluency is dramatically decreasing, at which time the pattern is distinct enough for probable PPA.

Semantic Dementia (Aphasia)

This variety was separated from PPA as 'semantic dementia' by Snowden et al. [12]. These patients progressively lose the meaning of words, but retain fluency and are able to carry out a conversation, so initially they are not obviously aphasic. Soon the impaired comprehension of nouns becomes evident and distinguishes the syndrome from other progressive difficulty naming objects. The picture is similar to 'transcortical sensory aphasia' in which articulation, phonology and syntax remain intact but the patient does not comprehend well and has word finding difficulty. Typically they ask the meaning of words they hear in conversation or asked about: 'what is broccoli?' Semantic substitutions are frequent and later fluent semantic jargon, often totally irrelevant to the questions asked or the topics discussed appear. They can not read some irregular words, because reading by meaning is lost, but they continue to read phonologically. In about half of the cases, visual and tactile agnosia is evident, in other words the loss is 'amodal' and not restricted to language. Patients with semantic dementia differ significantly from the fluent aphasics of AD because they have a relatively preserved episodic and autobiographical memory at least initially. Furthermore, AD patients tend not have the comprehension problem so prominently at earlier stages of illness. The behavior can be so bizarre that some of these patients are considered hysterical. Semantic dementia is often associated with bvFTD, and patients presenting with the behavioral symptoms often have elements of semantic dementia. Severe dominant side temporal atrophy is characteristic [13].

Corticobasal Degeneration/Progressive Supranuclear Palsy

The extrapyramidal component of PiD was recognized in the 1930s and later described as corticodentatonigral degeneration recognizing the similarity of the pathology to PiD [14]. These descriptions included language and behavioral changes, but the disease was described in movement disorder clinics subsequently under the label corticobasal degeneration [15]. The clinical syndrome of unilateral rigidity, prominent apraxia, gaze palsy, reflex myoclonus and the alien hand syndrome was emphasized and the cortical symptoms remained in the background until recently. There were some case reports describing patients presented clinically as CBD, but turned out to have Pick bodies or other FTD pathology [16]. Other cases pathologically typical of CBD have FTD or PPA without the extrapyramidal features [17]. We suggested that the clinical syndrome of prominent apraxia, unilateral extrapyramidal syndrome and alien hand phenomenon should be designated as corticobasal degeneration syndrome and CBD should be used for the pathological picture. (CBS is another abbreviation for the clinical syndrome.) Corticobasal degeneration syndrome showed significant overlap with the syndromes of FTD/Pick complex [18].

The syndrome of axial dystonia, bradykinesia, falls, dysphagia, and vertical gaze palsy was described as progressive supranuclear palsy (PSP) [19], but the overlap with CBD has been increasingly recognized [20]. Many CBD patients also have vertical gaze palsy; some have falls, and symmetrical extrapyramidal syndrome. PSP may follow FTD and PPA and vice versa in sufficient number of cases that the relationship is now considered well established. Some studies comparing the neuropsychological features of PSP and CBD found no significant difference between them [21]. The pathological biochemical and genetic evidence also support the relationship. There is continuing controversy to what extent PSP and CBD can be differentiated, and many still consider them separate disease entities but the evidence is in favor that CBD/PSP is also part of the Pick complex.

Motor Neuron Disease and FTD

Recently, a great deal of interest has been shown in the association of dementia with MND. Cognitive and behavioral impairment has been observed in amyotrophic lateral sclerosis (ALS), and some estimate it to be as high as 50% [22] and sometimes FTD or PA is observed. There are also some (about 10%) of cases of FTD and PPA that develop MND [23]. It also became evident that the majority of FTD and PPA cases (not only those with MND) have ubiquitin-positive, tau-negative inclusions in the cortex, which have been previously described in the motor neurons in ALS [24]. A new protein abnormality designated as TDP-43 was found to be common to both the ubiquinated variety of FTLD (FTLD-U) and ALS (see below).

Investigation

Although the clinical diagnosis is well within the competence of the general neurologist, psychiatrist and geriatrician, confirmation and support should be obtained in all cases with neuroimaging. In addition, a behavioral inventory and cognitive tests, especially language examination, are useful.

Neuroimaging preferably with MRI will quickly provide the diagnostic confirmation of focal atrophy in the majority of cases and it is essential to exclude a neoplasm, vasculitis and demyelinating disease. At times, CT is quite adequate for the purpose, but atrophy is more difficult to distinguish with CT. At times, subtle focal differences are unreported by general radiologists and a personal review of the scan is advisable. HMPO-SPECT and PET scanning may be more sensitive to focal change than structural imaging and amyloid or transmitter scanning may be used in the future.

Caregiver responses to a questionnaire, such as the Frontal Behavioral Inventory [25], used at the initial interview, turns out to be the most useful diagnostic tool for bv-FTD. The inventory was designed as a series of structured questions scripted so both the normal and abnormal aspects of the behaviors were included. Each item was scored on a scale of 4: 0 = none, 1 = mild or occasional, 2 = moderate, 3 = severe or most of the time. The items were grouped as negative behaviors such as apathy, aspontaneity, indifference, inflexibility, personal neglect, distractibility, inattention, loss of insight, logopenia, verbal apraxia, questioning the meaning of words and alien hand. These last four items were included to capture specific motor and speech behaviors, which may be associated with FTD. The positive group of behaviors contained items of disinhibition such as perseveration, irritability, jocularity, irresponsibility, inappropriateness, impulsivity, hoarding, restlessness, aggression, hyperorality and hypersexuality. A score above 30 is in the range for bvFTD. We demonstrated in a study with the behavioral inventory that using cognitive tests only 75% of FTD and AD patients can be distinguished, while adding FBI to the discriminant function 100% discrimination was achieved [25].

Neuropsychological deficits have been variable because of the types and methods of patient selection at different stages of illness and the tests used [26, 27]. Orientation and episodic memory is relatively preserved and the Mini-Mental Status Examination may be normal in early cases. Frontal lobe functions are impaired; however, some patients with behavioral presentation perform well on 'frontal' tests especially if they are seen early. Although FTD can present as a 'dysexecutive syndrome', frontal lobe or executive deficits are often involved in AD as well. Some preservation of memory is typical, but not universal by any means. There is often a memory complaint in FTD, but the reason for impaired memory performance could be related to inattention, lack of motivation and/or language impairment. Although drawings in FTD patients may be impoverished due to amotivational performance, visuospatial function is generally intact. Some patients may be perseverative in drawing. At times, copying can be compulsively faithful to detail. Visuospatial tasks requiring executive function, such as trail making, are impaired at an early stage, but block design and Raven's Coloured Progressive Matrices may be preserved. At times, impulsivity, disinhibition, perseveration, echopraxia and utilization behavior are observed during neuropsychological testing. In later stages, the patient may be too restless or language impaired to test.

Genetic testing yields a relatively high number of tau [28] and progranulin [29] mutations, although in only about 10% of the familial cases, and it is not widely available. The clinical phenotypes do not predict the pathology or the genotype with certainty, although the association of bvFTD with semantic dementia suggests ubiquitin-positive pathology and progranulin mutations (FTLD-U); the combination of CBD/PSP with PPA is likely associated with tau-positive pathology and tau mutation (FTLD-T) in the familial cases [30]. Other mutations such as the CHMP on chromosome 3 [31] and the valosin-containing protein on chromosome 9 [32] are infrequent. The TDP-43 protein [33] is more ubiquitous, but mutations were found on chromosome 1, only in ALS patients so far [34].

Glossary

1. Frontotemporal Dementia (FTD)
Used for both
A. The behavioral presentation, and
B. The overall disease.

2. Frontotemporal Degeneration (FTD)
A. Used for all pathological variants.
B. The abbreviation is the same as clinical FTD.

3. Frontotemporal Lobar Degeneration (FTLD)
A. Lobar was added for the overall pathological designation to reserve FTD for the behavioral presentation.
B. Also used for the overall clinical disease.

4. Pick's Disease (PiD)
A. The overall clinical syndrome, used less now, because of restricting it to 2.
B. Histologically defined entity, diagnosable only on post-mortem, with silver and tau-positive, round or oval inclusions in the cortex.

5. Pick Complex (FTD/Pick)
Includes all the clinical syndromes and underlying pathological variants. FTD/Pick is also used throughout this chapter combining 1 and 5 as a composite abbreviation.

6. Primary Progressive Aphasia (PPA)
Slowly progressive aphasia before anything else develops. This presenting syndrome is also part of FTD/Pick. It also has a variety of pathologies just like FTD. At times specified as progressive nonfluent aphasia (PNFA).

7. Semantic Dementia (SD)
A multimodality loss of meaning, difficulty with both comprehension and naming, especially nouns with preserved fluency.

8. Corticobasal Degeneration Syndrome (CBDS)
Unilateral rigidity, immobility, apraxia, and the 'alien hand', but many of these patients develop features of FTD and PPA. It overlaps with PSP (10).

9. Corticobasal Degeneration (CBD)
Basal ganglionic and cortical silver and tau-positive neuronal inclusions, often look like Pick bodies, 'Pick cells' are characteristic. Also used as the clinical syndrome (like in 8).

10. Progressive Supranuclear Palsy (PSP)
Defined by vertical gaze palsy, slowness, falling and dysarthria. The symptoms, pathology, tau biochemistry, and genetics overlap with CBDS (8) and CBD (9). Probably part of Pick complex. Some prefer to keep it separate.

11. FTD with Motor Neuron Disease (FTD-MND)
This was initially described as a clinical entity. Same as ALS-dementia.

12. FTD- with Motor Neuron Disease Inclusion Type of Pathology (FTD-MND, MNDID, FTLD-U)
Many cases of FTD with ubiquitin positive tau-negative inclusions, typical of MND, but most have no clinical MND. Also called motor neuron disease inclusion dementia (MNDID).

13. FTDP-17
FTD and parkinsonism linked to chromosome 17. Less than half of these families have tau mutations. The first published family also had amyotrophy (MND).

14. Dementia Lacking Distinctive Histology (DLDH)
Pathology without Pick bodies or typical CBD features. Most of these turn out to have MND type inclusions when stained with ubiquitin.

References

1 Pick A: Über die Beziehungen der senilen Hirnatrophie zur Aphasie. Prag Med Wochenschr 1892;17:165–167.
2 Gustafson L: Frontal lobe degeneration of non-Alzheimer type II. Clinical picture and differential diagnosis. Arch Gerontol Geriatr 1987;6:209–223.
3 The Lund and Manchester Groups: Clinical and neuropathological criteria for frontotemporal dementia. J Neurol Neurosurg Psychiatry 1994;57: 416–418.
4 Mesulam M-M: Primary progressive aphasia – differentiation from Alzheimer's disease. Ann Neurol 1987;22:533–534.
5 Kertesz A, Hudson L, Mackenzie IRA, et al: The pathology and nosology of primary progressive aphasia. Neurology 1994;44:2065–2072.
6 Neary D, Snowden JS, Gustafson L, et al: Frontotemporal lobar degeneration – a consensus on clinical diagnostic criteria. Neurology 1998;51: 1546–1554.
7 Gregory CA, Hodges JR: Frontotemporal dementia: use of consensus criteria and prevalence of psychiatric features. Neuropsychiatry Neuropsychol Behav Neurol 1996;9:145–153.
8 Cummings JL, Duchen LW: Kluver-Bucy syndrome in Pick disease: clinical and pathologic correlations. Neurology 1981;31:1415–1422.
9 Grossman M, Mickanin J, Onishi C et al: Progressive nonfluent aphasia, language, cognitive and PET measures contrasted with probable Alzheimer's disease. J Cog Neurosci 1996;8:135–154.
10 Cohen L, Benoit N, Van Eeckhout P, Ducarne B, Brunet P: Pure progressive aphemia. J Neurol Neurosurg Psychiatry 1993;56:923–924.
11 Weintraub S, Rubin NP, Mesulam M-M: Primary progressive aphasia: longitudinal course, neuropsychological profile, and language features. Arch Neurol 1990;47:1329–1335.
12 Snowden JS, Goulding PJ, Neary D: Semantic dementia: a form of circumscribed cerebral atrophy. Behav Neurol 1989;2:167–182.
13 Hodges JR, Patterson K, Oxbury S, Funnell E. Semantic dementia: progressive fluent aphasia with temporal lobe atrophy. Brain 1992;115:1783–1806.
14 Rebeiz JJ, Kolodny EH, Richardson EP Jr: Corticodentatonigral degeneration with neuronal achromasia. Arch Neurol 1968;18:20–33.
15 Gibb WRG, Luthert PJ, Marsden CD: Corticobasal degeneration. Brain 1989;112:1171–1192.
16 Lang AE, Bergeron C, Pollanen MS, Ashby P: Parietal Pick's disease mimicking cortical-basal degeneration. Neurology 1992;44:1436–1440.
17 Lippa CF, Smith TW, Fontneau N: Corticonigral degeneration with neuronal achromasia. A clinicopathological study of two cases. JNS 1990;98: 301–310.
18 Kertesz A, Martinez-Lage P, Davidson W, Munoz DG: The corticobasal degeneration syndrome overlaps progressive aphasia and frontotemporal dementia. Neurology 2000;55:1368–1375.
19 Steele JC, Richardson JC, Olszewski J: Progressive supranuclear palsy. Arch Neurol 1964;10:333–359.
20 Josephs KA, Petersen RC, Knopman DS, et al: Clinicopathologic analysis of frontotemporal and corticobasal degenerations and PSP. Neurology 2006;66:41–48.

21 Pillon B, Blin J, Vidailhet M, et al: The neuropsychological pattern of corticobasal degeneration: comparison with progressive supranuclear palsy and Alzheimer's disease. Neurology 1995;45: 1477–1483.

22 Lomen-Hoerth C, Anderson T, Miller B: The overlap of amyotrophic lateral sclerosis and frontotemporal dementia. Neurology 2002;59:1077–1079.

23 Neary D, Snowden JS, Mann DMA, Northen B, Goulding PJ, Macdermott N: Frontal lobe dementia and motor neuron disease. J Neurol Neurosurg Psychiatry 1990;53:23–32.

24 Munoz DG, Dickson DW, Bergeron C, Mackenzie IRA, Delacourte A, Zhukareva V: The neuropathology and biochemistry of frontotemporal dementia. Ann Neurol 2003;54(suppl 5):S24–S28.

25 Kertesz A, Davidson W, McCabe P, Munoz D: Behavioral quantitation is more sensitive than cognitive testing in frontotemporal dementia. Alzheimer Dis Assoc Disord 2003;17:223–229.

26 Miller BL, Cummings JL, Villanueva-Meyer J, et al: Frontal lobe degeneration: clinical, neuropsychological, and SPECT characteristics. Neurology 1991;41:1374–1382.

27 Hodges JR, Garrard P, Perry R, et al:. The differentiation of semantic dementia and frontal lobe dementia (temporal and frontal variants of frontotemporal dementia) from early Alzheimer's disease: a comparative neuropsychological study. Neuropsychology 1999;13:31–40.

28 Hutton M, Lendon CL, Rizzu P, et al: Association of missense and 5'-splice-site mutations in tau with the inherited dementia FTDP-17. Nature 1998;393: 702–705.

29 Baker M, Mackenzie IR, Pickering-Brown SM: Mutations in progranulin cause tau-negative frontotemporal dementia linked to chromosome 17. Nature 2006;442:916–919.

30 Kertesz A, Blair M, McMonagle P, Munoz DG: The diagnosis and course of frontotemporal dementia. Alzheimer Dis Assoc Disord 2007;21:155–163.

31 Skibinski G, Parkinson NJ, Brown JM, et al: Mutation in the endosomal ESCRT-III complex subunit CHMP2B in frontotemporal dementia. Nat Genet 2005;37:806–808.

32 Watts GD, Wymer J, Kovach MJ, et al: Inclusion body myopathy associated with Paget disease of bone and frontotemporal dementia is caused by mutant valosin-containing protein. Nat Genet 2004; 36:377–381.

33 Neumann M, Sampathu DM, Kwong LK, et al: Ubiquitinated TDP-43 in frontotemporal lobar degeneration and amyotrophic lateral sclerosis. Science 2006;314:130–133.

34 Sreedharan J, Blair IP, Tripathi VB et al: TDP-43 mutations in familial and sporadic amyotrophic lateral sclerosis. Science 2008;319:1668-1672.

Prof. Andrew Kertesz, MD FRCP(C)
University of Western Ontario, St. Joseph's Hospital
268 Grosvenor St., London, ON, N6A 4V2 (Canada)
Tel. +1 519 646 6032, Fax +1 519 646 6226, E-Mail andrew.kertesz@sjhc.london.on.ca

Giannakopoulos P, Hof PR (eds): Dementia in Clinical Practice.
Front Neurol Neurosci. Basel, Karger, 2009, vol 24, pp 149–159

Neuropathological Spectrum of Frontal Lobe Dementias

Enikö Kövari

Division of Neuropsychiatry, Department of Psychiatry, Geneva School of Medicine, Chêne-Bourg, Geneva, Switzerland

Abstract

Frontotemporal dementia (FTD) is characterized by different severity of frontotemporal atrophy, and histologically by neuronal loss, gliosis and spongiosis. Due to the new discoveries in biochemistry, genetics and neuropathology, re-examination of the former neuropathological criteria was necessary. Actually, we distinguish subgroups on the basis of the presence or absence of intraneuronal or intraneuronal and glial inclusions: the so-called FTD tauopathies, such as Pick's disease, corticobasal degeneration, progressive supranuclear palsy, FTD with parkinsonism linked to chromosome 17, argyrophilic grain disease and neurofibrillary tangle dementia. FTD nontauopathies include dementia lacking distinctive histology (without any known inclusion) and FTD (clinically with or without motor neuron disease) with ubiquitin-immunoreactive inclusions. In the latter group, a new pathological protein, the TAR-binding protein (TDP-43), was recently described as the main component of inclusion, and several new mutations were also discovered. The new neuropathological criteria could be a great help in the neuropathological diagnosis and in further clinicopathological studies, and the new discoveries are useful in understanding the underlying disease processes.

The clinical syndromes of frontotemporal dementia (FTD), semantic dementia, primary progressive nonfluent aphasia, and progressive apraxia called frontotemporal lobar dementia (FTLD) [1] regroup a diversity of neuropathological entities. With exception of genetically determined cases, a postmortem examination of the brain is necessary to obtain the definitive diagnosis of the underlying degenerative disease.

The gross examination of the brain in most cases reveals frontal and/or temporal – sometimes asymmetric – lobar atrophy. In early stages the brain could be normal, in advanced disease the severe atrophy may affect also the basal ganglia [2]. In cases with associated parkinsonism, loss of pigmentation of the substantia nigra is seen [3]. The common histological features are neuronal loss, spongiosis and cortical astrogliosis.

The clinical and neuropathological classifications have changed several times since the original description of the clinical entity by Arnold Pick in 1892 [4] and the underlying neuropathological changes by Alois Alzheimer in 1911 [5].

The classical neuropathological classification of FTD, earlier called Pick's disease (PiD), is based on histological hallmarks. After recognizing that the main histological feature, the Pick bodies (PiB), is present only in the minority of cases, Constantinidis et al. [6] determined 3 neuropathological subtypes: type A with PiB; type B with ballooned neurons (the so-called Pick cells) and type C, without any specific histological lesions. With the beginning of application of immunohistochemical methods in the 1980s, the Lund and Manchester Groups reclassified the FTD on the basis of the presence or absence and immunohistochemical patterns of intracellular inclusions. The frontal lobe degeneration type showed milder neuronal loss and spongiosis in the superficial cortical layers without intraneuronal inclusions; the Pick type was characterized by more severe neuronal loss and gliosis with or without PiB and swollen neurons, and in the motor neuron disease (MND) type ubiquitin-reactive inclusions were present in the involved areas [7].

Following the advances in molecular genetics, biochemistry and immunohistochemistry, a revision of the already existing neuropathological criteria was necessary. Corticobasal degeneration (CBD) and progressive supranuclear palsy (PSP) were classified as members of the subgroup of FTD tauopathies, and in the last years more and more genes (as the genes of TAR DNA-binding protein, *TDP-43,* on chromosome 1; valosin-containing protein, *VCP,* on chromosome 9p21-p12; progranulin, *PGRN,* on chromosome 17q21–22) were identified as having a possible role in the FTD with ubiquitin-reactive inclusions [8]. In 2001, the Work Group on Frontotemporal Dementia and Pick's Disease [9], and in 2007 the Midwest Consortium for Frontotemporal Lobar Degeneration [10] reviewed new discoveries in this field. The novel classification is based on the presence or absence of intracellular inclusions and, if present, on the biochemical composition of the pathological protein and genetic alterations (table 1). Thus, two main forms of FTD are distinguished: FTD tauopathies and FTD nontauopathies.

Frontotemporal Dementia Tauopathies (Frontotemporal Dementia with Tau-Immunoreactive Inclusions)

The main histological hallmark of this group is the presence of tau immunoreactive inclusions in the neurons and/or glial cells (astrocytes and oligodendrocytes). Tau is a microtubule-associated protein tau *(MAPT)* gene product with six tau isoforms in the human adult brain. Three isoforms contain three microtubule-binding repeats (3R), the others four (4R). On this basis, this group is divided into 3R, 4R and 3R and 4R subgroups.

Table 1. Classification of FTDs[1]

Tauopathies

1. Predominantly 3R tau-containing inclusions
   A. FTLD with PiB (PiD)
   B. FTLD with *MAPT* mutation (FTDP-17T)
2. Predominantly 4R tau-containing inclusions
   A. CBD
   B. PSP
   C. AgD
3. 3R and 4R tau-containing inclusions
   Neurofibrillary tangle dementia

Nontauopathies

1. FTLD without tau- or ubiquitin/P62-positive inclusions (dementia lacking distinctive histologic features, DLDH)
2. FTD-U ubiquitin-positive/P62-positive, tau-negative inclusions
   A. TDP-43 proteinopathies
      FTLD-U with or without MND (FTLD-U types 1–3)
      FTLD-U with *PGRN* mutation (FTLD-U type 3)
      FTLD-U with *VCP* mutation (FTLD-U type 4)
      FTLD-U linked to chromosome 9p (FTLD-U type 2)
   B. Non-TDP-43 proteinopathies
   - Ubiquitin and P62-positive, TDP-43 and tau-negative inclusions:
      FTLD-U with CHMP2B mutation
      BIBD
   - Ubiquitin, P62 and α-internexin-positive inclusions:
      NIFID

[1]Modified and simplified version based on reference [10].

Predominantly 3R Tauopathies

Pick's Disease

The term PiD was used for a long time for the entity that today is called FTD, but it became evident that cases showing the main histological feature, the PiB, are relatively rare, less than 20% of all FTD cases [11]; however, we do not have real epidemiological data.

Genetic predisposition of the PiD is not clear; it appears that most cases originally described as familial PiD are in reality FTDP-17 cases [12], considering that both have some similarities in their histological and immunohistochemical appearance.

In classical cases, the brain shows severe atrophy ('knife edge' type) of the frontal and/or temporal lobes. The posterior 1/3 of the temporal cortex and the peri-Rolandic area is typically spared (fig. 1a). The head of the caudate nucleus is flattened, and secondary to the brain and basal ganglia atrophy the anterior horns of the lateral ventricles are enlarged.

Neuronal loss, gliosis and spongiosis (fig. 1b) – depending on the severity – could affect only the superficial cortical layers or be transcortical. The main histological feature are PiBs, argyrophilic and tau-immunoreactive intracytoplasmic neuronal inclusions seen in the dentate gyrus (fig. 1c), subiculum, CA1 sector of hippocampus and layers II–III (and in severe cases also in layer VI) of the temporal and frontal neocortex and sometimes in several subcortical nuclei such as the caudate nucleus, thalamus, amygdala [13]. PiBs are spherical, well delimited, on hematoxylin-eosin staining basophilic inclusions situated in the cytoplasm of neurons [14].

Frontotemporal Dementia and Parkinsonism Linked to Chromosome 17

It has been known since 1986, that the *MAPT* gene is localized on chromosome 17. The identification of association of the *tau* gene mutations and FTDP-17T in 1994 [15] demonstrated that tau dysfunction itself could cause neurodegenerative disease [16]. The prevalence and incidence of FTDP-17T are unknown. Until the end of 2007, 39 mutations in 115 families were identified [8].

FTDP-17T shows an autosomal dominant inheritance affecting equally males and females. The average age at onset is 49 years [16]. It presents macroscopically with mild to severe frontal and/or temporal – sometimes asymmetric – atrophy, affecting also the caudate nucleus, putamen, globus pallidus, amygdala, hippocampus, ventral thalamus, substantia nigra and locus coeruleus [3,16].

The main histological characteristic is the presence of tau-immunoreactive inclusions in neurons or in both neurons and glial cells. The histological picture may vary depending on the type of *tau* gene mutation; however, there is some uniformity concerning the distribution of lesions. The alterations are seen in both the cortex and subcortical gray and white matter. Unspecific histological signs (seen in all forms of FTD): neuronal loss, gliosis, spongiosis are mostly transcortical. Argyrophilic, tau-immunoreactive inclusions are present in the neurons, oligodendrocytes and less commonly astrocytes of the affected regions. Cases without glial inclusions resemble PiD [8].

Predominantly 4R Tauopathies

Corticobasal Degeneration

The first description of CBD dates back to 1967 [17]. It is a member of the group of atypical parkinsonism. The prevalence is not known, but it is probably often underdiagnosed. Most cases are sporadic; however, in some familial CBD cases reported earlier, it remains to be determined whether they really correspond to FTDP-17T cases [16].

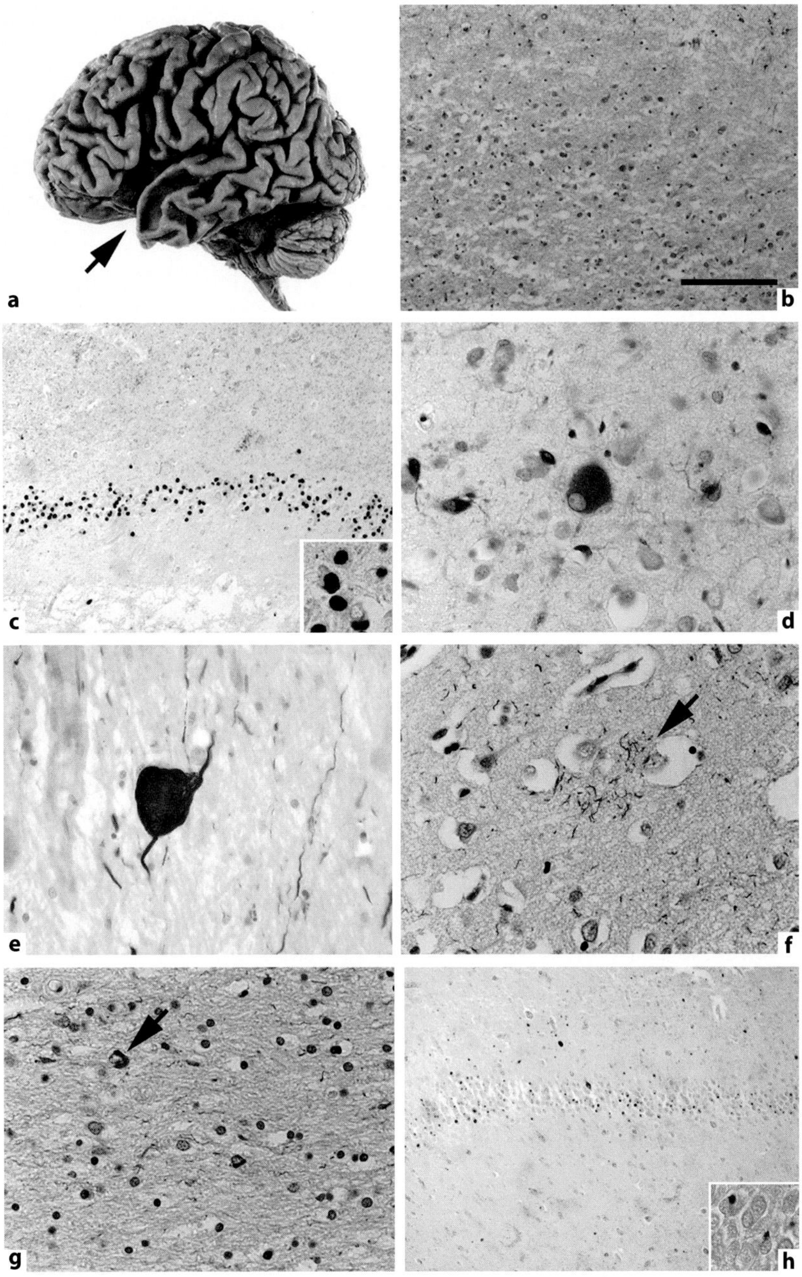

Fig. 1. **a**. Frontotemporal atrophy in PiD. Note the 'knife edge' atrophy of the anterior 2/3 of the superior temporal gyrus (arrow). **b** Spongiosis, neuronal loss and gliosis in the temporal cortex in PiD. **c** PiBs in the dentate gyrus in PiD. **d** Ballooned neurons in the anterior cingulate cortex. **e** Globoid NFT in the locus coeruleus. **f** Neuropil threads (arrow). **g** Coiled body in CBD (arrow). **h** Ubiquitin positive inclusions in the dentate gyrus in FTD-U. **b** Hematoxylin-eosin staining. **c, e** Tau-immunohistochemistry. **d** αB-crystallin immunohistochemistry. **f, g** Gallyas staining. **h** Ubiquitin immunohistochemistry. Scale bar: 200 μm (**b, c, h**); 50 μm (**d, e, f, g** and inserts **c** and **h**).

Classic CBD cases show focal, usually asymmetric cortical atrophy most pronounced in the peri-Rolandic region [18]. Brain stem atrophy is generally less severe than in PSP. On histological examination in the affected regions – mainly the peri-Rolandic region – cortical atrophy is seen due to the neuronal loss and gliosis, accompanied by spongiosis of the superficial layers. Swollen neurons (ballooned neurons) are present in the third, fifth and sixth cortical layers (fig. 1d) of the anterior cingulate cortex, insular cortex, superior frontal cortex, superior temporal cortex and also in the amygdala and claustrum [16, 19]. Ballooned neurons resemble Pick cells of PiD and show immunoreactivity for αB-crystallin. Tau-immunoreactive inclusions in the affected cortical areas have a pleomorph structure, they could be small and round resembling PiD or have a more filamentous or granular structure. Neurofibrillary tangles (NFTs) of the brainstem (substantia nigra and locus coeruleus) are globoid and they are called corticobasal bodies (fig. 1e). In addition to neurons, cell processes and glial cells are also affected in CBD. Neuropil threads and astrocytic plaques (tau-containing cell processes of neurons and astrocytes; fig. 1f) as well as coiled bodies (intracytoplasmic inclusions in oligodendrocytes; fig. 1g) are usually numerous in CBD [16].

Progressive Supranuclear Palsy (Steele-Richardson-Olszewski Disease)
PSP was first described in 1964 [20]. It is a sporadic disease; however, some familial cases with PSP-like phenotype are described. It presents typically with atypical parkinsonism and ophtalmoplegia, but early behavioral manifestations are not rare, rendering the distinction from FTD difficult [3]. True prevalence rates are not known, it is probably, as it is the case in CBD, underestimated.

The telencephalon generally does not show severe atrophy, but in most cases basal ganglia and brainstem are reduced in size and a discoloration of the substantia nigra and locus coeruleus is present. The main histological feature is the presence of tau-immunoreactive inclusions in neurons (globoid NFTs in the brainstem), glial cells (tufted thorn-shaped astrocytes), oligodendrocytes (coiled bodies) and neuropil threads. NFTs are numerous in the subthalamic nucleus, the basal ganglia and brainstem [18], and often the superior colliculus and oculomotor complex are also affected.

Argyrophilic Grain Disease
Argyrophilic grain disease (AgD) is a late-onset dementia described in 1987 by Braak and Braak [21]. For a long time, it was doubtful whether it represents a distinct entity, but later it was recognized that AgD is relatively frequent in the group of degenerative dementias. The prevalence varies between 5 and 10% in consecutive autopsy series [22].

On external examination, the brain appears normal; it shows at most a mild diffuse or frontotemporal atrophy and the hippocampus is generally preserved. The main histological hallmarks are the spindle-shaped argyrophilic, tau-containing grains in the neuronal processes and coiled bodies in oligodendrocytes. Argyrophilic grains are also present in cortical and subcortical structures, mainly in the transentorhinal and entorhinal cortex, followed by the amygdala and temporal cortex. High densities may be present also in the hypothalamic lateral tuberal nucleus. Coiled bodies, a nonspecific sign also present in other tauopathies such as CBD and PSP, are however always present in white matter close to the cortex. Ballooned neurons are a frequent feature in the amygdala [16, 22].

3R and 4R Tauopathies

Neurofibrillary Tangle Dementia (Tangle-Only Dementia)

Neurofibrillary tangle dementia, also called tangle-only dementia is mainly found in elderly individuals with a prevalence of 1.7–5.6% according to different autopsy series. The histological picture resembles Alzheimer's disease, the main hallmark is the presence of numerous NFTs in the hippocampus and parahippocampal regions, especially in the entorhinal and transentorhinal cortex, subiculum and the CA1 field of the hippocampus in the absence or scarcity of amyloid deposits (senile plaques) [23].

Frontotemporal Dementia Nontauopathies (Frontotemporal Dementia without Tau-Immunoreactive Inclusions)

Frontotemporal Lobar Degeneration

FTDL, called also dementia lacking distinctive histology (DLDH) represented until recently more than 50% of all FTD cases, but using immunohistochemistry more than 50% showed ubiquitin-reactive intracytoplasmic inclusions (FTLD-U) on reexamination [24]. In this group, both sporadic and familial cases are described [8]. On macroscopy, brains with DLDH show different severity of atrophy; histologically, only aspecific signs such as neuronal loss, gliosis and spongiosis are seen. Until today, no pathological protein has been identified that could play a role in DLDH.

FTD-U

The presence of ubiquitin-immunoreactive inclusion was originally described in MND with dementia [25]. Since this first description, a number of cases have been reported with ubiquitin-positive inclusions in the absence of MND in both sporadic and familial FTD [26, 27].

TDP-43 Proteinopathies

TDP-43, a nuclear protein, was recently identified as a major protein component of the ubiquitin-immunoreactive inclusions seen in sporadic and familial FTLD-U, with and without MND, and it is also present in sporadic amyotrophic lateral sclerosis, a form of MND [28,29]. The pathologic form of TDP-43 is hyperphosphorylated and ubiquitinated [29]. This subgroup seems to be the most frequent regarding all FTD cases [2, 30].

The ubiquitin and TDP-43 pathology represents a diversity of histological alterations: neuronal cytoplasmic inclusions (fig. 1h), neuronal intranuclear inclusions, dystrophic neurites, and glial cytoplasmic inclusions that are negative for tau, α-synuclein, β-amyloid, and neuronal intermediate filaments [31]. They are mostly present in the neurons of the dentate gyrus of the hippocampus and in the small neurons of the frontal and temporal cortices.

Depending on the location and type of inclusions, three histological patterns of ubiquitin inclusion pathology can be distinguished: (1) type 1, cases with a relative abundance of ubiquitin-positive pathology in superficial cortical layers and a predominance of long neuritic profiles over cytoplasmic inclusions; (2) type 2, cases with ubiquitin-positive pathology in both superficial and deep cortical layers with a predominance of cytoplasmic inclusions and only rare neuritic inclusions; (3) type 3, cases with a predominance of ubiquitin-positive pathology in superficial cortical layers and an abundance of cytoplasmic inclusions that are often ring shaped, short neuritic profiles, and ubiquitin-positive dots in the gray matter [32].

In the last years, several mutations were described in the familial forms of FTD-U as a cause of the degenerative disorder.

A mutation of the *PGRN* gene on chromosome 17 was described in cases FTD-U with mainly neuronal intranuclear inclusions, but also with neuronal cytoplasmic inclusions and dystrophic neurites. Interestingly, the ubiquinated pathological protein in these cases is not progranulin but TDP-43 [29].

VCP gene mutation presents as inclusion body myopathy associated with Paget's disease of bone and FTD, a rare autosomal dominant disease characterized by numerous neuronal intranuclear inclusions and few neuronal cytoplasmic inclusions and dystrophic neurites. The ubiquitinated protein also in these cases is TDP-43 [29].

In 2006, a novel mutation on chromosome 9 was described in a family with FTD-U [33].

These findings indicate that the *PGRN* and *VCP* gene mutations cause a loss or disturbed gene function, leading to impaired metabolism of TDP-43 [34]. Interestingly, the same pathological protein is found in the inclusion of familial cases without known mutation and also sporadic FTD-U cases.

Non-TDP-43 Proteinopathies

FTDL-U with CHMP2B Mutation. A rare cause of FTD linked to chromosome 3 is mutations in the charged multivesicular body protein 2B gene *(CHMP2B)* [35]. Brains show global (mostly) frontotemporal and central atrophy, with ubiquitin-positive but TDP-43- and tau-negative inclusions [36].

Basophilic Inclusion Body Disease. Until now, only about ten basophilic inclusion body disease (BIBD) cases have been reported. The young-onset dementia is associated with MND. The frontotemporal cortex, caudate nucleus, and substantia nigra are affected and histologically round cytoplasmic basophilic inclusions are seen immunonegative for tau, TDP-43 or neurofilaments. Inclusions are present in the basal ganglia and brainstem nuclei, in the motor neurons in the hypoglossal nuclei, and may be seen in the spinal anterior horn cells in cases with lower motor neuron signs and in lower numbers also in the hippocampus, subiculum, parahippocampal gyrus, amygdala, and cerebellar dentate nucleus [37].

Neuronal Intermediate Filament Inclusion Disease. The clinical and pathological characteristics of neuronal intermediate filament inclusion disease (NIFID) may resemble BIBD; however, in NIFID the frontal atrophy is more pronounced – mainly in its posterior part – compared to the temporal region. Histologically, with conventional stains, both disorders are indistinguishable, but in NIFID neuronal intracytoplasmic inclusions are neurofilament and α-internexin immunoreactive [37].

Conclusion

The exact neuropathological diagnosis of FTD has also clinical consequences. To make it, immunohistochemistry is necessary and commercially available antibodies are now available. In some forms, genetic counseling may be advisable.

References

1 Snowden J, Neary D, Mann D: Frontotemporal lobar degeneration: clinical and pathological relationships. Acta Neuropathol 2007;114:31–38.

2 Hodges JR, Davies RR, Xuereb JH, Casey B, Broe M, Bak TH, Kril JJ, Halliday GM: Clinicopathological correlates in frontotemporal dementia. Ann Neurol 2004;56:399–406.

3 Spillantini MG, Bird TD, Ghetti B: Frontotemporal dementia and parkinsonism linked to chromosome 17: a new group of tauopathies. Brain Pathol 1998;8: 387–402.

4 Pick A: Über die Beziehungen der senilen Hirnatrophie zur Aphasie. Prager Med Wochenschr 1892;17:165–167.

5 Alzheimer A: Über eignartige Krankheitsfalle des späteren Alters. Z Gesamte Neurol Psychiatr 1911; 4:378–388.

6 Constantinidis J, Richard J, Tissot R: Pick's disease. Histological and clinical correlations. Eur Neurol 1974;11:208–217.

7 The Lund and Manchester Groups: Clinical and neuropathological criteria for frontotemporal dementia. J Neurol Neurosurg Psychiatry 1994;57: 416–418.

8 Kumar-Singh S, Van Broeckhoven C: Frontotemporal lobar degeneration: current concepts in the light of recent advances. Brain Pathol 2007;17:104–114.

9 McKhann GM, Albert MS, Grossman M, Miller B, Dickson D, Trojanowski JQ: Clinical and pathological diagnosis of frontotemporal dementia: report of the work group on frontotemporal dementia and pick's disease. Arch Neurol 2001;58:1803–1809.

10 Cairns NJ, Bigio EH, Mackenzie IR, Neumann M, Lee VM, Hatanpaa KJ, White CL 3rd, Schneider JA, Grinberg LT, Halliday G, Duyckaerts C, Lowe JS, Holm IE, Tolnay M, Okamoto K, Yokoo H, Murayama S, Woulfe J, Munoz DG, Dickson DW, Ince PG, Trojanowski JQ, Mann DM: Neuropathologic diagnostic and nosologic criteria for frontotemporal lobar degeneration: consensus of the consortium for frontotemporal lobar degeneration. Acta Neuropathol 2007;114:5–22.

11 Rosso SM, Donker Kaat L, Baks T, Joosse M, de Koning I, Pijnenburg Y, de Jong D, Dooijes D, Kamphorst W, Ravid R, Niermeijer MF, Verheij F, Kremer HP, Scheltens P, van Duijn CM, Heutink P, van Swieten JC: Frontotemporal dementia in the netherlands: patient characteristics and prevalence estimates from a population-based study. Brain 2003;126:2016–2022.

12 Foster NL, Wilhelmsen K, Sima AA, Jones MZ, D'Amato CJ, Gilman S: Frontotemporal dementia and parkinsonism linked to chromosome 17: a consensus conference. Conference participants. Ann Neurol 1997;41:706–715.

13 Tsuchiya K, Ikeda K: Basal ganglia lesions in 'pick complex': a topographic neuropathological study of 19 autopsy cases. Neuropathology 2002;22:323–336.

14 Forno LS, Eng LF, Selkoe DJ: Pick bodies in the locus ceruleus. Acta Neuropathol 1989;79:10–17.

15 Wilhelmsen KC, Lynch T, Pavlou E, Higgins M, Nygaard TG: Localization of disinhibition-dementia-parkinsonism-amyotrophy complex to 17q21–22. Am J Hum Genet 1994;55:1159–1165.

16 Dickson DW, Bergeron C, Hauw J-J, Jellinger KA, Lantos P, Mizusawa H: Frontotemporal dementia and parkinsonism linked to chromosome 17 associated with tau gene mutations (FTDP-17T); in Dickson DW (ed): Neurodegeneration: The Molecular Pathology of Dementia and Movement Disorders. Basel, ISN Neuropath Press, 2003, pp 86–102.

17 Rebeiz JJ, Kolodny EH, Richardson EP Jr: Corticodentatonigral degeneration with neuronal achromasia: a progressive disorder of late adult life. Trans Am Neurol Assoc 1967;92:23–26.

18 Wakabayashi K, Takahashi H: Pathological heterogeneity in progressive supranuclear palsy and corticobasal degeneration. Neuropathology 2004;24:79–86.

19 Armstrong RA, Cairns NJ, Lantos PL: A quantitative study of the pathological lesions in the neocortex and hippocampus of twelve patients with corticobasal degeneration. Exp Neurol 2000;163:348–356.

20 Steele JC, Richardson JC, Olszewski J: Progressive supranuclear palsy. A heterogeneous degeneration involving the brain stem, basal ganglia and cerebellum with vertical gaze and pseudobulbar palsy, nuchal dystonia and dementia. Arch Neurol 1964;10:333–359.

21 Braak H, Braak E: Argyrophilic grains: characteristic pathology of cerebral cortex in cases of adult onset dementia without Alzheimer changes. Neurosci Lett 1987;76:124–127.

22 Tolnay M, Clavaguera F: Argyrophilic grain disease: a late-onset dementia with distinctive features among tauopathies. Neuropathology 2004;24:269–283.

23 Yamada M: Senile dementia of the neurofibrillary tangle type (tangle-only dementia): neuropathological criteria and clinical guidelines for diagnosis. Neuropathology 2003;23:311–317.

24 Kövari E, Gold G, Giannakopoulos P, Bouras C: Cortical ubiquitin-positive inclusions in frontotemporal dementia without motor neuron disease: a quantitative immunocytochemical study. Acta Neuropathol 2004;108:207–212.

25 Okamoto K, Hirai S, Yamazaki T, Sun XY, Nakazato Y: New ubiquitin-positive intraneuronal inclusions in the extra-motor cortices in patients with amyotrophic lateral sclerosis. Neurosci Lett 1991;129:233–236.

26 Kertesz A, Kawarai T, Rogaeva E, St George-Hyslop P, Poorkaj P, Bird TD, Munoz DG: Familial frontotemporal dementia with ubiquitin-positive, tau-negative inclusions. Neurology 2000;54:818–827.

27 Kövari E, Leuba G, Savioz A, Saini K, Anastasiu R, Miklossy J, Bouras C: Familial frontotemporal dementia with ubiquitin inclusion bodies and without motor neuron disease. Acta Neuropathol 2000;100:421–426.

28 Arai T, Hasegawa M, Akiyama H, Ikeda K, Nonaka T, Mori H, Mann D, Tsuchiya K, Yoshida M, Hashizume Y, Oda T: TDP-43 is a component of ubiquitin-positive tau-negative inclusions in frontotemporal lobar degeneration and amyotrophic lateral sclerosis. Biochem Biophys Res Commun 2006;351:602–611.

29 Neumann M, Sampathu DM, Kwong LK, Truax AC, Micsenyi MC, Chou TT, Bruce J, Schuck T, Grossman M, Clark CM, McCluskey LF, Miller BL, Masliah E, Mackenzie IR, Feldman H, Feiden W, Kretzschmar HA, Trojanowski JQ, Lee VM: Ubiquitinated TDP-43 in frontotemporal lobar degeneration and amyotrophic lateral sclerosis. Science 2006;314:130–133.

30 Mackenzie IR, Shi J, Shaw CL, Duplessis D, Neary D, Snowden JS, Mann DM: Dementia lacking distinctive histology (DLDH) revisited. Acta Neuropathol 2006;112:551–559.

31 Mackenzie IR, Baker M, Pickering-Brown S, Hsiung GY, Lindholm C, Dwosh E, Gass J, Cannon A, Rademakers R, Hutton M, Feldman HH: The neuropathology of frontotemporal lobar degeneration caused by mutations in the progranulin gene. Brain 2006;129:3081–3090.
32 Sampathu DM, Neumann M, Kwong LK, Chou TT, Micsenyi M, Truax A, Bruce J, Grossman M, Trojanowski JQ, Lee VM: Pathological heterogeneity of frontotemporal lobar degeneration with ubiquitin-positive inclusions delineated by ubiquitin immunohistochemistry and novel monoclonal antibodies. Am J Pathol 2006;169:1343–1352.
33 Vance C, Al-Chalabi A, Ruddy D, Smith BN, Hu X, Sreedharan J, Siddique T, Schelhaas HJ, Kusters B, Troost D, Baas F, de Jong V, Shaw CE: Familial amyotrophic lateral sclerosis with frontotemporal dementia is linked to a locus on chromosome 9p13.2–21.3. Brain 2006;129:868–876.
34 Cairns NJ, Neumann M, Bigio EH, Holm IE, Troost D, Hatanpaa KJ, Foong C, White CL 3rd, Schneider JA, Kretzschmar HA, Carter D, Taylor-Reinwald L, Paulsmeyer K, Strider J, Gitcho M, Goate AM, Morris JC, Mishra M, Kwong LK, Stieber A, Xu Y, Forman MS, Trojanowski JQ, Lee VM, Mackenzie IR: TDP-43 in familial and sporadic frontotemporal lobar degeneration with ubiquitin inclusions. Am J Pathol 2007;171:227–240.
35 Skibinski G, Parkinson NJ, Brown JM, Chakrabarti L, Lloyd SL, Hummerich H, Nielsen JE, Hodges JR, Spillantini MG, Thusgaard T, Brandner S, Brun A, Rossor MN, Gade A, Johannsen P, Sorensen SA, Gydesen S, Fisher EM, Collinge J: Mutations in the endosomal ESCRTIII-complex subunit CHMP2B in frontotemporal dementia. Nat Genet 2005;37:806–808.
36 Holm IE, Englund E, Mackenzie IR, Johannsen P, Isaacs AM: A reassessment of the neuropathology of frontotemporal dementia linked to chromosome 3. J Neuropathol Exp Neurol 2007;66:884–891.
37 Yokota O, Tsuchiya K, Terada S, Ishizu H, Uchikado H, Ikeda M, Oyanagi K, Nakano I, Murayama S, Kuroda S, Akiyama H: Basophilic inclusion body disease and neuronal intermediate filament inclusion disease: a comparative clinicopathological study. Acta Neuropathol 2008;115:561–575.

Enikö Kövari, MD
Division of Neuropsychiatry, Department of Psychiatry
Geneva School of Medicine, 2, chemin du Petit-Bel-Air
CH–1225 Chêne-Bourg, Geneva (Switzerland)
Tel. +1 41 22 305 53 61, Fax +41 22 305 53 50, E-Mail eniko.kovari@hcuge.ch

Giannakopoulos P, Hof PR (eds): Dementia in Clinical Practice.
Front Neurol Neurosci. Basel, Karger, 2009, vol 24, pp 160–167

Frontotemporal Dementia Neuroimaging: A Guide for Clinicians

William W. Seeley

Department of Neurology, University of California, San Francisco, and UCSF Memory and Aging Center, San Francisco, Calif., USA

Abstract

Frontotemporal dementia represents an important cause of dementia that requires differentiation from Alzheimer's disease. As molecular therapies for both diseases begin to emerge, neuroimaging biomarkers will be needed that can improve diagnostic accuracy and enable treatment monitoring. At present, structural magnetic resonance imaging provides a useful adjunct to clinical assessment, helping to distinguish frontotemporal dementia from Alzheimer's disease and from nonneurodegenerative disease. Future imaging research will seek to more directly assay disease by assessing network level pathophysiology and accumulation of misfolded proteins in cerebral tissues.

Neuroimaging plays an increasing role in the differential diagnosis of dementia. This chapter outlines the utility, challenges, and promise of neuroimaging tools, emphasizing the role these techniques can play in distinguishing frontotemporal dementia (FTD) from Alzheimer's disease (AD).

Each dementia syndrome features a signature pattern of functional anatomic impairment associated with a short differential diagnosis of underlying histopathologies (table 1). Therefore, careful assessment for regional atrophy patterns can lead the clinician to the most likely disease. Advanced structural-functional connectivity mapping techniques, such as diffusion tensor imaging (DTI) and functional connectivity magnetic resonance imaging (fcMRI), may further extend clinicians' reach by allowing us to probe endpoints closely related to neurodegeneration pathophysiology. But no longer must we think of neuroimaging as only a measure of brain structure and function. Molecular imaging promises to help us peer deeper, into the specific microscopic pathomolecular substrates of disease. This capability, once fully developed, has the potential to overcome some of the most vexing challenges in dementia differential diagnosis.

Table 1. AD and FTD functional and anatomical impairments

Syndrome	Early deficit	Early network/ region	Underlying histopathology
Typical AD	episodic memory	MTL-PCC/precuneus-lateral temporoparietal	AD, rarely FTLD-U with hippocampal sclerosis
FTD			
BvFTD	social-emotional function	R > L ACC-FI, frontal pole, amygdala, striatum	FTLD-T = FTLD-U[1], rarely AD
SD	semantic knowledge or emotional meaning	L or R temporal pole, amygdala, sACC, FI	FTLD-U[1] >> FTLD-T = AD
PNFA	motor speech and language fluency	L inferior frontal cortex, precentral insula, striatum	FTLD-T > FTLD-U[1] > AD
FTD-MND	social-emotional function, motor power	ACC-FI network, bulbar and spinal motor nuclei > primary motor cortex	FTLD-MND[1]

L = Left; MTL = medial temporal lobe; R= right; sACC = subgenual ACC.
[1]Usually with TDP-43-immunoreactive neuronal cytoplasmic inclusions.

Frontotemporal Dementia Clinical-Anatomic Features

AD and FTD are the leading causes of dementia in patients under 65 years of age [1]. FTD refers to a group of dissociable neurodegenerative syndromes that impair social behavior, speech, language, or a combination of these faculties. In contrast to typical amnestic AD, which leads to predominant medial temporal and posterior cortical atrophy, FTD involves specific anterior brain structures often spared in AD (table 1; fig. 1) [2, 3]. Three major FTD clinical subtypes are recognized [4]. In the behavioral variant (bvFTD), early symptoms include disinhibition, apathy, compulsivity and overeating, and loss of sensitivity to others' emotions, accompanied by progressive degeneration within anterior brain regions, including anterior cingulate (ACC) and adjacent rostromedial prefrontal cortex (rmPFC), the frontal insula (FI), frontal pole, and ventral striatum [2, 5]. Dorsolateral prefrontal cortex degeneration occurs later [6], accompanied by executive functioning deficits often absent at earlier stages. In semantic dementia (SD), a fluent aphasia that erodes word, object, and emotional meaning [7, 8], patients show temporal pole degeneration followed by ventromedial prefrontal cortex, subgenual ACC, FI, and ventral striatal involvement [8, 9]. SD often follows an asymmetric pattern but rapidly proceeds to involve homologous contralateral structures [8, 9]. Progressive nonfluent aphasia (PNFA), in contrast, leads to dysfluent, effortful, agrammatic speech and dominant frontal operculum, supplementary motor area, and dorsal insula atrophy [10, 11]. The consistency of these syndromic regional atrophy patterns has helped structural MRI become a useful adjunct

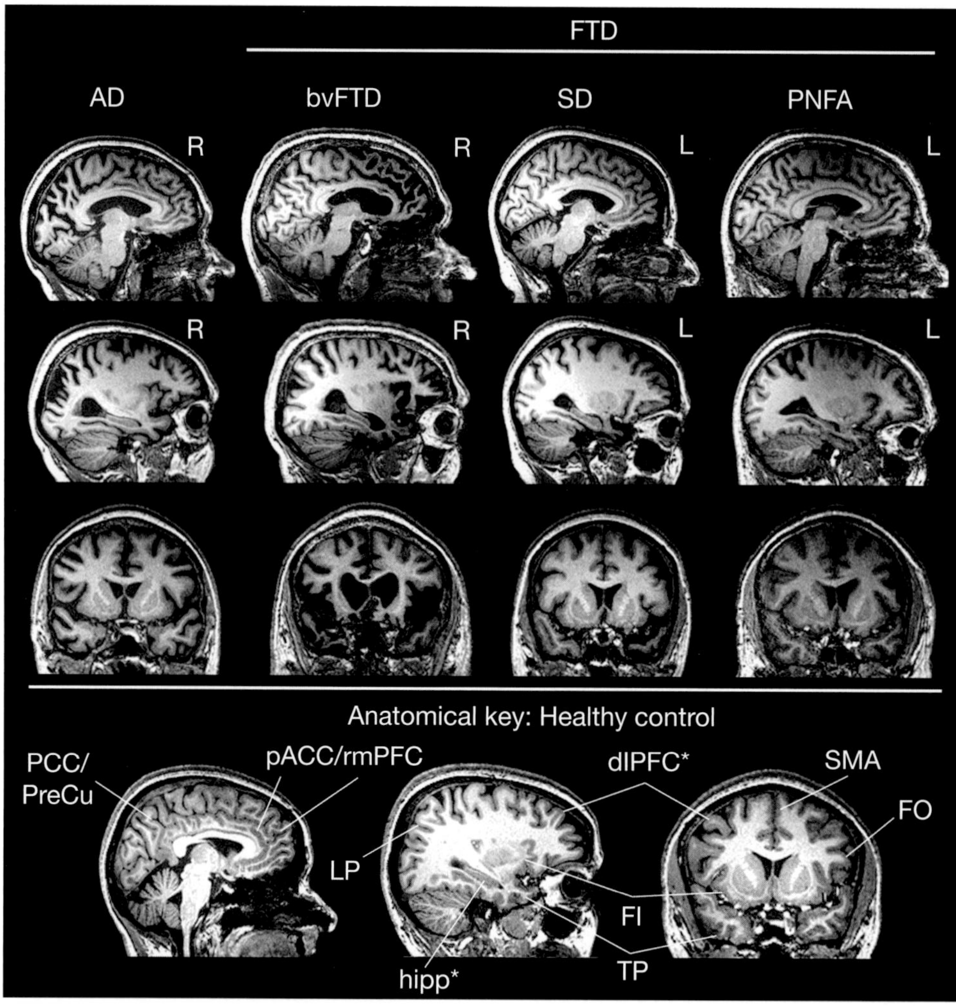

Fig. 1. Practical approach to T1-weighted structural MRI in patients with FTD and AD. Evaluation of sagittal (adjacent to the midline and through the circular insular sulcus) and coronal (at the level of the temporal poles) slices can help differentiate AD from FTD subtypes. In AD, prominent atrophy in posterior cingulate/precuneus (PCC/preCu) and lateral parietal (LP) regions stands in contrast to sparing of pregenual ACC (pACC)/rmPFC and FI. BvFTD shows the opposite pattern, devastating ACC/rmPFC/FI and sparing PCC/preCu/LP. SD features marked often asymmetric temporal pole (TP) atrophy, and PNFA reflects dominant frontal operculum (FO) and supplementary motor area (SMA) degeneration. Comparable slices from a healthy control subject (bottom) provide an anatomical index. *Note that hippocampus (hipp) and dorsolateral prefrontal cortex (dlPFC) atrophy often fail to differentiate AD from FTD syndromes, especially in early age-at-onset patients. In the coronal images, the right side of the image corresponds to the left side of the brain.

to the symptoms, signs, and neuropsychological features that define each syndrome. A practical approach to differentiating FTD syndromes from each other and AD is outlined in figure 1.

Challenges in Frontotemporal Dementia Neuroimaging

Early and Magnetic Resonance-Negative Frontotemporal Dementia

While the broad FTD functional and regional deficit profiles have now been well characterized [12], much less is known about early stage and preclinical disease. Most patients present to academic centers more than 5 years after symptom onset, making it difficult to study large early-stage cohorts. Previously, we used voxel-based morphometry to identify regions atrophied in 15 patients with very mild bvFTD, defined as a Clinical Dementia Rating score of 0.5 [6]. Intriguingly, rather than showing any single region of focal atrophy, early bvFTD featured circumscribed degeneration within a 'network' of frontal paralimbic and subcortical regions bearing known anatomical connections in primates. Still, much controversy surrounds what to do when the scan is normal. In some bvFTD series, nearly half of all patients presented with little or no MR-detectable atrophy [13, 14]. Some patients with minimal atrophy evolved into a progressive bvFTD syndrome, but others showed no progression over long-term follow-up, suggesting that they were misdiagnosed on clinical grounds. Positron emission tomography may prove more sensitive to frontotemporal dysfunction [15, 16], but hypometabolism is also less specific to neurodegenerative disease than atrophy, raising the potential for false-positive diagnoses among psychiatric bvFTD mimickers. fcMRI and DTI have been proposed as potential early disease alternatives to traditional MRI [17, 18], and could prove the most sensitive and specific for early bvFTD neurodegeneration, but these modalities remain unproven. In contrast to bvFTD, SD and PNFA routinely show focal atrophy at presentation [14], suggesting that these diagnoses should be made with caution when neuroimaging studies are unremarkable.

Predicting Pathology

A primary goal of clinical syndromic diagnosis is to guide pathological predictions. So far, however, such efforts have been disappointing. BvFTD, for example, relates equally to tau-positive frontotemporal lobar degeneration (FTLD-T) and tau-negative, ubiquitin-positive pathology (FTLD-U) [19]. Prediction accuracy improves for SD and PNFA, but remains challenging, and up to a third of these patients may show underlying AD at autopsy [20, 21]. The basic principle giving rise to these observations is that molecular histopathologies do not follow set rules about which brain systems to target. Rather, despite important, indeed defining anatomical predilections, neurodegenerative diseases can make their way inside one of several networks to cause disease. This flexibility should not surprise us, as AD has long been known to cause diverse clinical syndromes, including visual, motor, language, and even behavioral variants [20, 22, 23]. Accordingly, even if emerging structural-functional techniques make good biomarkers, helping to detect and follow early-stage FTD, these methods may not overcome pathological differential diagnostic hurdles. Pinpointing an affected system with neuroimaging may never be enough to predict pathology with the accuracy required; rather, we may need to image the misfolded proteins themselves.

Structural MRI will remain the front-line modality for ruling out nondegenerative (vascular, infectious, demyelinating, and neoplastic) mimickers of neurodegenerative disease. Accurate molecular diagnosis will become paramount, however, once disease-specific treatments emerge. Since patients with SD, PNFA, and even bvFTD can show AD pathology at autopsy [20], and because structural MRI reflects the clinical syndrome rather than pathology, molecular imaging may soon become a necessary clinical supplement to guide treatment decisions. A molecular approach, like amyloid imaging with the Pittsburgh compound-B [24], will have two major goals in this context. First, we must prevent FTLD patients from receiving potentially toxic AD therapies from which they are unlikely to benefit. Second, we need a mechanism to know exactly which 20–30% of clinical FTD patients have senile plaques and neurofibrillary tangles, not FTLD, throughout their networked anterior brain structures [25]. Eventually, imaging tools to distinguish FTLD-T from FTLD-U will be needed if divergent treatments for these FTLD subtypes can be brought to the clinic.

Mixed Pathology

Pathological admixtures within FTD syndromes add an additional challenge. Recent studies suggest that bvFTD can relate to mixed FTLD-T and FTLD-U pathology [26], suggesting that some patients may someday benefit from treatments aimed at both tau and TDP-43 biology. Furthermore, dual AD and progressive supranuclear palsy pathology can mimic bvFTD, leading to clinical misdiagnosis [Seeley et al., unpubl. data]. This overlap underscores how important it will become to integrate clinical findings (e.g. motor and oculomotor signs) with molecular imaging results (e.g. positive Pittsburgh compound-B scan) in formulating final pathological predictions.

Role of Neuroimaging in Frontotemporal Dementia Research

Selective Vulnerability

Large-scale neuropathological studies including asymptomatic elders dying without dementia have helped to define a typical AD neuroanatomical progression [27], which begins with neurofibrillary tangle formation in layer 2 entorhinal cortex pyramidal neurons [28]. Similar approaches have been applied to define a staging system for Parkinson's disease [29]. A similar approach cannot be applied to FTLD, because this pathology is rarely found in unaffected individuals at autopsy. In this light, finding the regions and neurons first affected in FTD requires an in vivo approach. We have used the bvFTD anatomical pattern as a roadmap for exploring cell-specific pathology in autopsy materials [30]. Similar approaches to SD and PNFA pathology may reveal selectively vulnerable neurons within the temporal poles (SD) or frontal operculum (PNFA) that incite the neurodegenerative cascade throughout the network that progressively succumbs to produce each full-blown syndrome. Studies of these vulnerable neurons, moreover, may help shed new light on disease pathogenesis.

Clinical Biomarkers to Help Find Treatments

The molecular biology of FTD has witnessed major recent advances, including the discovery of TDP-43, the disease protein underlying most FTLD-U [31], and progranulin, the gene linked to inherited FTLD-U [32]. This progress has raised hopes for FTD treatments within the coming decades. Imaging has the potential to play an important role in the development of such treatments, providing a biologically robust but noninvasive clinical biomarker. Potential modalities for disease monitoring include quantitative MRI, positron emission tomography, fcMRI, and DTI. With new approaches and refinements coming forth at a rapid pace, the prospects for a useful imaging biomarker seem bright.

Conclusion

FTD has emerged as an important cause of dementia and a tractable subject for scientific study. Neuroimaging has defined the anatomy of the disease, begun to elucidate lesion-deficit correlations, and contributes to syndromic differential diagnosis. Further developed, neuroimaging could become a key player in the race to treat and cure FTD.

References

1 Ratnavalli E, Brayne C, Dawson K, Hodges JR: The prevalence of frontotemporal dementia. Neurology 2002;58:1615–1621.

2 Varrone A, Pappata S, Caraco C, Soricelli A, Milan G, Quarantelli M, Alfano B, Postiglione A, Salvatore M: Voxel-based comparison of rCBF SPET images in frontotemporal dementia and Alzheimer's disease highlights the involvement of different cortical networks. Eur J Nucl Med Mol Imaging 2002; 29:1447–1454.

3 Rabinovici GD, Seeley WW, Kim EJ, Gorno-Tempini ML, Rascovsky K, Pagliaro TA, Allison SC, Halabi C, Kramer JH, Johnson JK, Weiner MW, Forman MS, Trojanowski JQ, Dearmond SJ, Miller BL, Rosen HJ: Distinct MRI atrophy patterns in autopsy-proven Alzheimer's disease and frontotemporal lobar degeneration. Am J Alzheimers Dis Other Demen 2007;22:474–488.

4 Neary D, Snowden JS, Gustafson L, Passant U, Stuss D, Black S, Freedman M, Kertesz A, Robert PH, Albert M, Boone K, Miller BL, Cummings J, Benson DF: Frontotemporal lobar degeneration: a consensus on clinical diagnostic criteria. Neurology 1998; 51:1546–1554.

5 Rosen HJ, Gorno-Tempini ML, Goldman WP, Perry RJ, Schuff N, Weiner M, Feiwell R, Kramer JH, Miller BL: Patterns of brain atrophy in frontotemporal dementia and semantic dementia. Neurology 2002, 58:198–208.

6 Seeley WW, Crawford R, Rascovsky K, Kramer JH, Weiner M, Miller BL, Gorno-Tempini ML: Frontal paralimbic network atrophy in very mild behavioral variant frontotemporal dementia. Arch Neurol 2008;65:249–255.

7 Snowden J, Goulding P, Neary D: Semantic dementia: a form of circumscribed cerebral atrophy. Behav Neurol 1989;2:167–182.

8 Seeley WW, Bauer AM, Miller BL, Gorno-Tempini ML, Kramer JH, Weiner M, Rosen HJ: The natural history of temporal variant frontotemporal dementia. Neurology 2005;64:1384–1390.

9 Brambati SM, Rankin KP, Narvid J, Seeley WW, Dean D, Rosen HJ, Miller BL, Ashburner J, Gorno-Tempini ML: Atrophy progression in semantic dementia with asymmetric temporal involvement: a tensor-based morphometry study. Neurobiol Aging 2007; Epub ahead of print.

10 Gorno-Tempini ML, Dronkers NF, Rankin KP, Ogar JM, Phengrasamy L, Rosen HJ, Johnson JK, Weiner MW, Miller BL: Cognition and anatomy in three variants of primary progressive aphasia. Ann Neurol 2004;55:335–346.

11 Josephs KA, Duffy JR, Strand EA, Whitwell JL, Layton KF, Parisi JE, Hauser MF, Witte RJ, Boeve BF, Knopman DS, Dickson DW, Jack CR Jr, Petersen RC: Clinicopathological and imaging correlates of progressive aphasia and apraxia of speech. Brain 2006;129:1385–1398.

12 Schroeter ML, Raczka K, Neumann J, Yves von Cramon D: Towards a nosology for frontotemporal lobar degenerations-a meta-analysis involving 267 subjects. Neuroimage 2007;36:497–510.

13 Davies RR, Kipps CM, Mitchell J, Kril JJ, Halliday GM, Hodges JR: Progression in frontotemporal dementia: identifying a benign behavioral variant by magnetic resonance imaging. Arch Neurol 2006; 63:1627–1631.

14 Kipps CM, Davies RR, Mitchell J, Kril JJ, Halliday GM, Hodges JR: Clinical significance of lobar atrophy in frontotemporal dementia: application of an MRI visual rating scale. Dement Geriatr Cogn Disord 2007;23:334–342.

15 Diehl-Schmid J, Grimmer T, Drzezga A, Bornschein S, Riemenschneider M, Forstl H, Schwaiger M, Kurz A: Decline of cerebral glucose metabolism in frontotemporal dementia: a longitudinal 18F-FDG-PET-study. Neurobiol Aging 2007;28:42–50.

16 Foster NL, Heidebrink JL, Clark CM, Jagust WJ, Arnold SE, Barbas NR, DeCarli CS, Turner RS, Koeppe RA, Higdon R, Minoshima S: FDG-PET improves accuracy in distinguishing frontotemporal dementia and Alzheimer's disease. Brain 2007; 130:2616–2635.

17 Greicius MD, Srivastava G, Reiss AL, Menon V: Default-mode network activity distinguishes Alzheimer's disease from healthy aging: evidence from functional MRI. Proc Natl Acad Sci USA 2004; 101:4637–4642.

18 Borroni B, Alberici A, Premi E, Archetti S, Garibotto V, Agosti C, Gasparotti R, Di Luca M, Perani D, Padovani A: Brain magnetic resonance imaging structural changes in a pedigree of asymptomatic progranulin mutation carriers. Rejuven Res 2008;11: 585–595.

19 Hodges JR, Davies RR, Xuereb JH, Casey B, Broe M, Bak TH, Kril JJ, Halliday GM: Clinicopathological correlates in frontotemporal dementia. Ann Neurol 2004;56:399–406.

20 Alladi S, Xuereb J, Bak T, Nestor P, Knibb J, Patterson K, Hodges JR: Focal cortical presentations of Alzheimer's disease. Brain 2007;130:2636–2645.

21 Mesulam M, Wicklund A, Johnson N, Rogalski E, Leger GC, Rademaker A, Weintraub S, Bigio EH: Alzheimer and frontotemporal pathology in subsets of primary progressive aphasia. Ann Neurol 2008; 63:709–719.

22 Hof PR, Bouras C, Constantinidis J, Morrison JH: Balint's syndrome in Alzheimer's disease: specific disruption of the occipito-parietal visual pathway. Brain Res 1989;493:368–375.

23 Johnson J, Head E, Kim R, Starr A, Cotman C: Clinical and pathological evidence for a frontal variant of Alzheimer disease. Arch Neurol 1999;56:1233–1239.

24 Klunk WE, Engler H, Nordberg A, Wang Y, Blomqvist G, Holt DP, Bergstrom M, Savitcheva I, Huang GF, Estrada S, Ausen B, Debnath ML, Barletta J, Price JC, Sandell J, Lopresti BJ, Wall A, Koivisto P, Antoni G, Mathis CA, Langstrom B: Imaging brain amyloid in Alzheimer's disease with Pittsburgh Compound-B. Ann Neurol 2004;55:306–319.

25 Rabinovici GD, Furst AJ, O'Neil JP, Racine CA, Mormino EC, Baker SL, Chetty S, Patel P, Pagliaro TA, Klunk WE, Mathis CA, Rosen HJ, Miller BL, Jagust WJ: 11C-PIB PET imaging in Alzheimer disease and frontotemporal lobar degeneration. Neurology 2007;68:1205–1212.

26 Freeman SH, Spires-Jones T, Hyman BT, Growdon JH, Frosch MP: TAR-DNA binding protein 43 in Pick disease. J Neuropathol Exp Neurol 2008;67:62–67.

27 Braak H, Braak E: Neuropathological staging of Alzheimer-related changes. Acta Neuropathol 1991; 82:239–259.

28 Hyman BT, Damasio AR, Van Hoesen GW, Barnes CL: Alzheimer's disease: cell-specific pathology isolates the hippocampal formation. Science 1984;298: 83–95.

29 Braak H, Ghebremedhin E, Rub U, Bratzke H, Del Tredici K: Stages in the development of Parkinson's disease-related pathology. Cell Tissue Res 2004; 318:121–134.

30 Seeley WW, Carlin DA, Allman JM, Macedo MN, Bush C, Miller BL, Dearmond SJ: Early frontotemporal dementia targets neurons unique to apes and humans. Ann Neurol 2006;60:660–667.

31 Neumann M, Sampathu DM, Kwong LK, Truax AC, Micsenyi MC, Chou TT, Bruce J, Schuck T, Grossman M, Clark CM, McCluskey LF, Miller BL, Masliah E, Mackenzie IR, Feldman H, Feiden W, Kretzschmar HA, Trojanowski JQ, Lee VM: Ubiquitinated TDP-43 in frontotemporal lobar degeneration and amyotrophic lateral sclerosis. Science 2006;314:130–133.

32 Baker M, Mackenzie IR, Pickering-Brown SM, Gass J, Rademakers R, Lindholm C, Snowden J, Adamson J, Sadovnick AD, Rollinson S, Cannon A, Dwosh E, Neary D, Melquist S, Richardson A, Dickson D, Berger Z, Eriksen J, Robinson T, Zehr C, Dickey CA, Crook R, McGowan E, Mann D, Boeve B, Feldman H, Hutton M: Mutations in progranulin cause tau-negative frontotemporal dementia linked to chromosome 17. Nature 2006;442:916–919.

Prof. William W. Seeley, MD
University of California, San Francisco
UCSF Memory and Aging Center, Box 1207
San Francisco, CA 94143-1207 (USA)
Tel. +1 415 476 2793, Fax +1 415 476 4800, E-Mail wseeley@memory.ucsf.edu

Giannakopoulos P, Hof PR (eds): Dementia in Clinical Practice.
Front Neurol Neurosci. Basel, Karger, 2009, vol 24, pp 168–178

Frontotemporal Dementia: Therapeutic Interventions

Mario F. Mendez

David Geffen School of Medicine at UCLA, and Neurobehavior V.A. Greater Los Angeles Healthcare System, Los Angeles, Calif., USA

Abstract

The management of frontotemporal dementia (FTD), a disorder characterized by varied behavioral symptoms, primarily involves the use of psychoactive medications. Although there are no approved treatments for the disorder, selective serontonin receptor inhibitors, such as sertraline, paroxetine, or fluoxetine, can decrease disinhibition-impulsivity, repetitive behaviors, and eating disorders in FTD. Low doses of trazodone or an atypical antipsychotic such as aripriprazole can also help manage significantly disturbed or agitated behavior. The acetylcholinesterase inhibitors used for patients with Alzheimer's disease have not had significant efficacy for patients with FTD, but memantine, another dementia medication, is under investigation for the treatment of this disorder. In addition to drug therapy, the nonpharmacological management of patients with FTD focuses on education, behavioral interventions, and care of the caregivers. Most recently, investigators have initiated steps toward rational drug therapy with the development of outcome measures for clinical drug trials in FTD and the characterization of treatment targets such tau protein or the TAR DNA-binding protein 43. This approach holds great promise for an eventual treatment for this devastating early-onset dementia.

Frontotemporal dementia (FTD), or the behavioral variant frontotemporal lobar degeneration, is a common early-onset disorder [1, 2]. FTD is probably the third most common neurodegenerative dementia after Alzheimer's disease (AD) and dementia with Lewy bodies (DLB). The average age at onset of FTD is 56–58 years, and FTD accounts for at least 20% of dementia patients with disease onset of less than 65 years [1]. Given its usual early onset and frequency, FTD tends to afflict people in the prime of life, when they may be at their most productive holding jobs and providing for families. Consequently, FTD has a disproportionate impact on families and society.

Despite the significance and impact of FTD, there are no approved treatments for the disorder, and there are no completed double-blind, randomized, controlled clinical trials in FTD. The development of drug therapy is difficult, in part because of the varied behavioral nature of this disorder. The main manifestations of FTD are alterations in personality and behaviors, including apathy, disinhibition, disturbed social behavior, decreased empathy, loss of insight and self-referential behavior, repetitive and compulsive behaviors, and changes in oral and dietary behavior [2]. These behavioral symptoms result in frequent misdiagnoses, clinical diagnostic criteria that are difficult to apply, and no proven measures for monitoring FTD patients [3]. Until recently, there were no instruments demonstrated to be useful in measuring outcomes in clinical drug trials [4].

Given the lack of specific treatments for FTD, clinicians charged with the management of these patients have resorted to several overlapping strategies (table 1). First, they have applied treatments and interventions used for patients with AD. Second, they have been interested in targeting neurotransmitter deficits in FTD, similar to the use of acetylcholinesterase inhibitors (ChEIns) for AD. Third, they have treated the behavioral symptoms of FTD with psychoactive medications used for psychiatric disorders. Only in the last 2 years, with the revolution in the understanding of the basic science of FTD, have we begun to develop true rational drug interventions based on an understanding of the underlying pathophysiology [5].

In addition to drug therapy, there are a range of nonpharmacological interventions that can ameliorate the impact of this disorder. Most of these are derived from an extensive experience in managing patients with dementia in general; however, some nonpharmacological interventions are specific to FTD. These nonpharmacological measures focus on education, behavioral management strategies, and caregiver support.

Alzheimer's Disease Therapies in FTD

ChEIns have attained wide use in the treatment of patients with AD. Drugs such as donepezil, rivastigmine, or galantamine can improve memory measures, temporarily improve cognition, and stabilize daily functioning among AD patients [6]. ChEIns may even ameliorate the noncognitive behavioral manifestations of AD [7, 8], suggesting that they could benefit patients with FTD as well. ChEIns have had specific effects on apathy or indifference, disinhibition, anxiety, depression, agitation, and the emergence of aberrant motor behavior [6–9]. In addition, neuropsychiatric symptoms in AD subjects who demonstrate FTD-like frontal lobe perfusion deficits on single photon emission tomography have responded to ChEIns therapy, particularly with decreased disinhibition and irritability [10]. In the absence of medications for FTD, it is, therefore, not surprising that many clinicians prescribe ChEIns in an attempt to treat these patients.

A few reports suggest improvement among patients with FTD treated with ChEIns [11, 12]. In a clinical report, Lampl et al. [11] described 9 FTD patients who had been treated with donepezil or rivastigmine for variable periods of time and found

Table 1. Pharmacological treatment of FTD[1]

1	Neuropsychiatric symptoms such as disinhibition-impulsivity, repetitive or stereotypical behaviors, and food or carbohydrate craving, may respond to SSRI and serotonergic agents such as sertraline, paroxetine, fluoxetine, or fluvoxamine. Start at low doses and increase gradually as needed.
2	Trazodone (beginning at 25 mg) can be effective for agitation as well as other neuropsychiatric behaviors. Somnolence limits its usefulness.
3	Marked disinhibition-impulsivity or aggressive and disruptive behaviors may respond to small doses of atypical antipsychotics such as aripripazole, but these medications should be avoided because of an increased risk of EPS.
4	ChEIns (donezepil, rivastigmine, galantamine) are of unclear benefit in FTD and could exacerbate disinhibition-impulsivity and repetitive or stereotypical behaviors.
5	The role of memantine as a neuroprotective agent in FTD is under investigation.
6	Antioxidants, e.g. vitamin E at 400–2,000 IU, may slow the progression of FTD.
7	Other drugs may target specific behaviors such as inappropriate sexuality and rapid eye movement behavior disorder. Parkinsonian symptoms have a modest response to dopaminergic agents. Psychostimulants or modafinil may help apathy-abulia. Carbamazepine, valproate, or lamotrigine may diminish long-term emotional fluctuations. These and other drugs await clinical trials in order to determine their efficacy in FTD.

[1]Modified from Mendez et al. [2].

improvement in the 4 males on general cognitive and single photon emission tomography measures. One open-label study compared 20 FTD patients treated with 3–9 mg/day of rivastigmine with 20 matched FTD controls after 12 months of follow-up [12]. The rivastigmine-treated group had a general amelioration of behavioral changes on the neuropsychiatric and caregiver measures. The FTD patients in this study, however, were older by about 10 years than the average age at onset for FTD and had uncharacteristically significant memory and other cognitive impairments, delusions, and hallucinations [12]. Although some conclude that this study reflects class II evidence of efficacy for ChEIns in FTD [13], the patient characteristics suggest that many of their 'FTD' patients may have had AD.

The rest of the available data does not provide convincing evidence that FTD patients benefit from medications that increase brain acetylcholine. First of all, unlike AD, in FTD there is no neuropathological evidence of a cholinergic deficit, such as cholinergic loss in the nucleus basalis of Meynert or abnormal choline acetyltransferase levels in the temporal poles [14, 15]. Secondly, more recent reports did not find clinical improvement from ChEIns among FTD patients. Using galantamine, Kertesz et al. [16] treated 36 patients with FTD and related syndromes in an 18-week, open-label phase and an 8-week randomized, placebo-controlled phase. They found no significant differences in behavior or language from galantamine. Mendez et al. [17] compared 12 FTD patients who received donepezil for 6 months with 12 FTD controls. The groups did not differ on most behavioral variables at baseline or at 6 months; however, the donepezil group had greater worsening than the non-donepezil group on the FTD Inventory measures of disinhibition and compulsive or stereotypical acts. The worsened behaviors abated after discontinuation of the medication.

Memantine, another AD medication, may have greater potential than ChEIns for the treatment of FTD patients. There is a rationale for the use of this putative neuroprotective agent in patients with FTD. Memantine is an NMDA receptor antagonist that prevents glutamine-mediated excitotoxic injury to neurons. One case series of 3 FTD patients noted improvement in neuropsychiatric symptoms, particularly in apathy, agitation, and anxiety [18]; otherwise, there is limited clinical evidence for the use of memantine for FTD. The drug, however, is sufficiently promising to have generated the first multicenter clinical trial for the treatment of FTD. A 26-week, placebo-controlled, randomized clinical trial of memantine for FTD and related syndromes has started with the goal of enrolling a total of 140 patients at 12 sites in North America [19].

Neurotransmitters and Therapy in Frontotemporal Dementia

The neurochemistry of FTD indicates roles for treatments aimed at the serotonergic and dopaminergic systems rather than the cholinergic system [14, 20]. In FTD, serotonergic $5HT_{1A}$ and $5HT_{2A}$ receptor levels are decreased in frontotemporal regions [14], and 40% of neurons are lost in the midbrain raphe nucleus, suggesting a presynaptic 5HT neuronal disturbance [21]. Cerebrospinal fluid (CSF) levels of 5-HIAA, the substrate of serotonin, are reduced among depressed FTD patients compared to AD patients [22]. Dopaminergic pathways are also affected in FTD [20]. CSF levels of homovanillic acid, the substrate for dopamine, are significantly lower in FTD subjects than in AD subjects [22]. Functional neuroimaging studies further show decreased binding of a dopamine D2 postsynaptic ligand in the superior frontal regions of subjects with FTD [23]. Finally, among 25 FTD patients, there was a strong correlation between CSF homovanillic acid/5HIAA ratios, a measure of serotonergic modulation of dopaminergic neurotransmission, and aggressive behavior [24].

Role of Psychoactive Medications

Patients with FTD often require psychoactive agents to treat their neuropsychiatric symptoms. Selective serotonergic reuptake inhibitors (SSRIs) or serotonergic transport inhibitors may allow FTD patients to compensate for the serotonergic deficits noted above. SSRIs such as fluoxetine, fluvoxamine, sertraline, and paroxetine can decrease disinhibition, repetitive or stereotypical behaviors, hyperorality, and sexually inappropriate behaviors among FTD patients [25–29]. In an early study, 4 of 5 FTD patients treated with fluoxetine, sertraline, or paroxetine for a minimum of 3 months demonstrated improvement in neuropsychiatric symptoms [25]. In another study, most FTD patients treated with sertraline had a decrease in their stereotypical movements [26]. Fluvoxamine also decreased stereotypical behaviors in a 12-week open label study of 16 FTD patients and in a case report of 2 others [30, 31]. Paroxetine has been successful in the treatment of repetitive, stereotypical behaviors in FTD [27, 32], and an open-label experience suggests that paroxetine may be helpful for the symptomatic management of this disorder [28]. In contrast, one randomized, placebo-controlled trial failed to show efficacy for paroxetine and instead noted impairments on learning tasks [33]. Other reports indicate that SSRIs can decrease the dietary changes of FTD, particularly the carbohydrate and food cravings [25], and diminish sexually inappropriate behavior and aggression [34].

Trazodone, a unique antidepressant that also inhibits serotonin reuptake, has been helpful in the management of agitation and other neuropsychiatric behaviors in FTD [27, 32]. In a randomized, placebo-controlled trial [35], trazodone was effective in treating the most disruptive behavioral symptoms of this disorder. Furthermore, a meta-analysis of SSRI and trazodone effects in FTD patients showed significant improvements in neuropsychiatric symptoms [29]. The somnolence associated with trazodone primarily limits its usefulness.

Behavioral symptoms refractory to SSRIs or trazodone may be responsive to atypical antipsychotic medications [36]. These newer antipsychotics have less dopamine D2 receptor occupancy and greater affinities for serotonin and noradrenaline receptors. Marked disinhibition, aggressive behavior, or verbal outbursts may respond to small doses of risperidone, clozapine, olanzapine, quetiapine, ziprasidone, or aripiprazole [19, 27, 37–39]. In an open-label study with a 24-month follow-up, 17 FTD patients had improved agitation, misconduct, and delusions and decreased caregiver distress on olanzapine [36].

Despite therapeutic benefit, clinicians should not routinely use antipsychotic medications, even the newer atypical antipsychotics, in FTD patients because of potential somnolence, weight gain, and, in particular, extrapyramidal side effects (EPS). Similar to patients with DLB, some FTD patients are especially vulnerable to EPS and tardive dyskinesias [40–42]. Also similar to DLB, in FTD there may be a failure to upregulate dopamine D2 receptors in response to postsynaptic receptor blockade. An early report found a unique tendency to moderate parkinsonism on therapeutic doses of haloperidol risperidone [40]. Subsequently, investigators described 24 patients with FTD and related syndromes who received antipsychotic medications [41]. Eight (33%) of these patients had side effects with 5 (21%) with severe EPS. Recently, antecollis, a rare form of tardive dystonia which can appear months after drug cessation, occurred in 3 FTD patients who received atypical antipsychotics (risperidone, clozapine, olanzapine, quetiapine, ziprasidone) [43]. Moreover, many of the behavioral problems of FTD are not clearly response to atypical antipsychotic medications [42]. Aripiprazole, which has partial agonistic properties at serotonin $5HT_{1A}$ and dopamine D2 receptors, could be an exception. A recent report of an FTD patient on aripiprazole showed stabilization of symptoms and improved frontal glucose metabolism on positron emission tomography after a month [44]. Nevertheless, clinicians need more information on aripiprazole before using it routinely in FTD.

Other Symptomatic Pharmacological Therapy

Clinicians and investigators have considered a number of other agents for treating the manifestations of FTD. Parkinsonian features in FTD show only a modest response to carbidopa/levodopa, amantadine, bromocryptine, or pramipexole [27, 32]. Behavioral disturbances, however, may improve with selegiline [45]. Meclobemide, a selective and reversible MAOA inhibitor, improved affect and decreased stereotypical behaviors and aggression in 6 FTD patients [46]. Preliminary reports with the psychostimulant methylphenidate suggest a possible beneficial effect on risk-taking behavior and on electroencephalograms in FTD [47, 48]. Drugs can target specific behaviors, such as conjugated estrogens or leupron for inappropriate sexual behavior among men and clonazepam for rapid eye movement behavior disorder in some FTD-parkinsonism patients. The antiepileptic mood stabilizers, valproate, carbamazepine, and lamotrigine, deserve further study as therapeutic agents in this disorder. In addition, limited reports among FTD patients have suggested beneficial effects of piracetam, idazoxan, gaunfacine, allopurinol, lithium plus SSRI, and even calcium EDTA [27, 37, 49]. Finally, many vitamins and supplements are often used for prevention, without proof of benefit [38]. Empirically, antioxidants such as vitamin E may slow the progression of FTD.

There have been specific attempts to treat the language disorders in the FTD-related syndromes of progressive nonfluent aphasia and semantic dementia. The main benefit is derived from a knowledgeable speech pathologist who can design a program of therapy tailored to the patient which includes traditional speech therapies, learning paradigms, and augmentative speech devices, where indicated. Attempts to treat progressive nonfluent aphasia with medications have yielded limited results. Bromocryptine and other dopaminergic agents, including buproprion, may improve some adynamic aspects of aphasia and are often worth a trial [50].

Future Disease-Modifying Treatments

Increased understanding of the pathophysiology of FTD may lead to promising compounds with therapeutic potential. Most patients with FTD have either a tauopathy or a TAR-DNA-binding protein (TDP-43) proteinopathy [5]. In the future, there may be specific disease-modifying treatments that alter abnormally phosphorylated tau residues or the expression of TDP-43 protein [5, 51, 52]. For example, lithium and valproate may decrease the accumulation of hyperphosphorylated tau proteins [51]. These drugs are inhibitors of glycogen synthase kinase 3b, which phosphorylates tau. The coadministration of lithium with SSRIs may have synergistic potential in treating FTD [48]. Other mechanisms to modulate total phospho-tau are those that inhibit heat-shock proteins, cyclin-dependent kinase 5, and fibrillization [5]. Additional experimental treatments include microtubular stabilizing agents such as paclitaxel and immunosuppressants such as FK506 [5]. Still, other therapies may target progranulin, a peptide growth factor that plays important roles in mediating neuronal development and inflammation. Research is just beginning into these and other potential disease-modifying agents for FTD.

In order to conduct clinical trials in FTD, there have to be well-characterized outcome measures, similar to those used in AD. Fortunately, a large, multicenter study of patients with FTD and related syndromes recently developed outcome measures for clinical trials in FTD [4]. Patients underwent neuropsychological, functional, behavioral, neurological and magnetic resonance imaging assessment at baseline and 12 months later. Two global measures, a modified Clinical Dementia Rating Scale (containing additional domains in behavior and language) and the Clinician's Global Impression of Change, demonstrated decline in the majority of patients. The neuropsychological tests combined into language and executive function composites were additionally sensitive to clinical changes in FTD. With these measures, the stage is now set for the initiation of more clinical trials for the treatment of FTD.

Nonpharmacological Therapy

Nonpharmacological interventions include education, behavioral management, and specific behavioral restrictions (table 2). Clinicians help caregivers by explaining that the neuropsychiatric features have a neurological basis [32]. Education on the fact that FTD alters personality characteristics and behavior can help caregivers accept and adjust to the patients' altered behavior. Behavioral management techniques can target socially disruptive behaviors, such as inappropriate commentary or touching, as well as stereotypical acts. One strategy is to redirect behaviors using the Antecedent-Behavior-Consequence Model aimed at modifying the antecedents or the consequences of the behavior [53]. Another strategy is to use rehabilitation techniques or retraining via their preserved procedural memory [54]. There often need to be specific restrictions to prevent access to food if overeating, to the outside if there is roaming, or to decision-making if there is poor judgment. When hyperorality is present, dietary restrictions and supervision are vital to preventing excessive weight gain or the dangerous placement of non-food items in the mouth [38]. Clinicians should evaluate FTD behaviors in terms of the threat to safety as well as frequency

Table 2. Nonpharmacological treatment of FTD[1]

1	Education-explanation on the nature of the disease and that the neuropsychiatric features have a neurological basis and are not 'deliberate' behaviors.
2	Behavioral management strategies and interventions, e.g. social misconduct and stereotypical behaviors may respond to diversion or, retraining, or other strategies.
3	Specific behavioral restrictions/certain behaviors require restructuring the environment, e.g. hyperorality, roaming, or compulsions. In particular, FTD patients lack judgment and require monitoring and restriction of decision making.
4	Attend to the patient's daily quality of life: mood status, social connectedness, ability to communicate, physical activity, and nutritional status.
5	Attend to functional issues: activities of daily living, home environment and safety, alternative transportation (FTD patients should not drive), independence vs. alternative living situations, and safe return bracelet.
6	Assure that the patient has a primary medical doctor.
7	Evaluate the need for genetic counseling, if other family members are affected.
8	Caring for caregiver: evaluate the need for family or caregiver psychological counseling as well as support groups, respite or relief including involvement of other family members, and referral to community resources, e.g. AD Caregivers Resource Center Caregiver Resource Center (www.caregiver.org) and the Association of Frontotemporal Dementias (www.ftd-picks.org)

[1]Modified from Mendez et al. [2].

and duration [55]. Finally, clinicians need to attend to the patients' quality of life, functional status (including interdicting driving), general medical needs, and, when indicated, appropriateness for genetic counseling.

FTD is very stressful to the caregiver and support of the family is critically important. Behavioral disturbances among FTD patients, such as apathy, disinhibition, mood disorders, and agitation, are particularly associated with high levels of caregiver distress. Caregivers may need support from other family members, counselors, and support groups and referrals to respite care and community resources. As FTD progresses, patients usually display increasing apathy and fewer intrusive behaviors such as disinhibition and stereotypical actions, which may result in easier behavioral management and correspondingly decreased caregiver stress [19].

Conclusions

Although there is no specific cure for FTD and related syndromes, several treatments are possible. Serotonin binding is decreased in FTD [29], and SSRIs such as sertraline, paroxetine, or fluoxetine can decrease disinhibition-impulsivity, repetitive and stereotypical behaviors, and overeating or carbohydrate craving [25–27]. Trazodone at low doses may be particularly helpful for agitated behavior. Marked disinhibition, aggressive behavior, or verbal outbursts may respond to small doses of atypical antipsychotics; however, caution is advised as some FTD patients have a hypersensitivity to these medications [40–42]. There is questionable benefit from ChEIns such as donezepil, rivastigmine, or galantamine [16, 17]; however, investigators are currently studying memantine as a treatment for FTD. The nonpharmacological management of patients with FTD focuses on education, behavioral interventions, and care of the caregivers. Finally, the recent, remarkable breakthroughs in the neuroscience of FTD hold the promise of disease-modifying therapies in the not too distant future.

References

1 Johnson JK, Diehl J, Mendez MF, et al: Frontotemporal lobar dementia: demographic characteristics of 353 patients. Arch Neurol 2005;62:925–930.

2 Mendez MF, Lauterbach EC, Sampson S, ANPA COR: The neuropsychiatry of frontotemporal dementia and related syndromes: a report by the ANPA Committee on Research. J Neuropsychiatry Clin Neurosci, in press.

3 Mendez MF, Perryman KM: Neuropsychiatric features of frontotemporal dementia. Evaluation of consensus criteria and review. J Neuropsychiatry Clin Neurosci 2002;14:424–429.

4 Knopman D, Boeve B, Caselli R, Graff-Radford NR, Kramer JH, Mendez MF, Miller BL: Longitudinal tracking of FTLD. Toward developing clinical trial methodology. Alzheimer Dis Assoc Disord 2007; 21:S58–S63.

5 Trojanowski JQ, Duff K, Fillit H, Koroshetz W, Kuret J, Murphy D, Refolo L: New directions for frontotemporal dementia drug discovery. Alzheimer Dem 2008;4:89–93.

6 Rogers SL, Farlow MR, Doody RS, Mohs R, Friedhoff LT: A 24-week, double-blind, placebo-controlled trial of donepezil in patients with Alzheimer's disease. Neurology 1998;50:136–145.

7 Trinh NH, Hoblyn J, Mohanty S, Yaffe K: Efficacy of cholinesterase inhibitors in the treatment of neuropsychiatric symptoms and functional impairment in Alzheimer's disease: a meta-analysis. JAMA 2003; 289:210–216.

8 Cummings JL, Schneider L, Tariot PN, Kershaw PR, Yuan W: Reduction of behavioral disturbances and caregiver distress by galantamine in patients with Alzheimer's disease. Am J Psychiatry 2004;161:532–538.

9 Holmes C, Wilkinson D, Dean C, et al: The efficacy of donepezil in the treatment of neuropsychiatric symptoms in Alzheimer disease. Neurology 2004;63: 214–219.

10 Mega MS, Dinov ID, Lee L, O'Connor SM, Masterman DM, Wilen B, Mishkin F, Toga AW, Cummings JL: Orbital and dorsolateral frontal perfusion defect associated with behavioral response to cholinesterase inhibitor therapy in Alzheimer's disease. J Neuropsychiatry Clin Neurosci 2000;12:209–218.

11 Lampl Y, Sadeh M, Lorberboym M: Efficacy of acetylcholinesterase inhibitors in frontotemporal dementia. Ann Pharmacother 2004;38:1967–1968.

12 Moretti R, Torre P, Antonello RM, Cattaruzza T, Cazzato G, Bava A: Rivastigmine in frontotemporal dementia: an open-label study. Drugs Aging 2004; 21:931–937.

13 Kessler H, Supprian T, Falkai P: Pharmacological treatment options in frontotemporal dementia. Fortschr Neurol Psychiatr 2007;75:714–719.

14 Procter AW, Qurne M, Francis PT: Neurochemical features of frontotemporal dementia. Dement Geriatr Cogn Disord 1999;10(suppl 1):80–84.

15 Sparks DL, Markesbery WR: Altered serotonergic and cholinergic synaptic markers in Pick's disease. Arch Neurol 1991;48:796–799.

16 Kertesz A, Morlog D, Light M, Blair M, Davidson W, Jesso S, Brashear R: Galantamine in frontotemporal dementia and primary progressive aphasia. Dement Geriatr Cogn Disord 2008;25:178–185.

17 Mendez MF, Shapira JS, McMurtray A, Licht E: Preliminary report: behavioral worsening on donepezil in patients with frontotemporal dementia. Am J Geriatr Psychiatry 2007;15:84–87.

18 Swanberg MM: Memantine for behavioral disturbances in frontotemporal dementia: a case series. Alzheimer Dis Assoc Disord 2007;21:164–166.
19 Boxer AL, Boeve BF: Frontotemporal dementia treatment: current symptomatic therapies and implications of recent genetic, biochemical, and neuroimaging studies. Alzheimer Dis Assoc Disord 2007;21:S79–S87.
20 Rinne JO, Laine M, Kaasinen V, Norvasuo-Heila MK, Nagren K, Helenius H: Striatal dopamine transporter and extrapyramidal symptoms in frontotemporal dementia. Neurology 2002;58:1489–1493.
21 Yang Y, Schmitt HP: Frontotemporal dementia: evidence for impairment of ascending serotoninergic but not noradeneregic innervation. Immunocytochemical and quantitative study using a graph method. Acta Neuropathol (Berl) 2001;101:256–270.
22 Sjogren M, Minthon L, Passant U, Blennow K, Wallin A: Decreased monoamine metabolites in frontotemporal dementia and Alzheimer's disease. Neurobiol Aging 1998;19:379–384.
23 Frisoni GB, Pizzolato G, Bianchetti A, Chierichetti F, Ferlin G, Battistin L, Trabucchi M: Single photon emission computed tomography with ^{99}Tc-HMPAO and ^{123}I-IBZM in Alzheimer's disease and dementia of frontal type: preliminary results. Acta Neurol Scand 1994;89:199–203.
24 Engelborghs S, Vloeberghs E, Le Bastard N, Van Buggenhout M, Mariën P, Somers N, Nagels G, Pickut BA, De Deyn PP: The dopaminergic neurotransmitter system is associated with aggression and agitation in frontotemporal dementia. Neurochem Int 2008;52:1052–1060.
25 Swartz JR, Miller BL, Lesser IM, Darby AL: Frontotemporal dementia: treatment response to serotonin selective reuptake inhibitors. J Clin Psychiatry 1997;58:212–216.
26 Mendez MF, Shapira JS, Miller BL: Stereotypical movements in frontotemporal dementia. Mov Disord 2005;20:742–745.
27 Chow TW: Frontotemporal dementias: clinical features and management. Semin Clin Neuropsychiatry 2003;8:58–70.
28 Moretti R, Torre P, Antonelli RM, Cazzato G, Bava A: Frontotemporal dementia: paroxetine as a possible treatment of behavior symptoms. A randomized, controlled, open 14-month study. Eur Neurol 2003;49:13–19.
29 Huey ED, Putnam KT, Grafman J: A systematic review of neurotransmitter deficits and treatments in frontotemporal dementia. Neurology 2006;66:17–22.
30 Ikeda M, Shigenobu K, Fukuhara R, Hokoishi K, Maki N, Nebu A, Komori K, Tanabe H: Efficacy of fluvoxamine as a treatment for behavioral symptoms in frontotemporal lobar degeneration patients. Dement Geriatr Cogn Disord 2004;17:117–121.
31 Ishikawa H, Shimomura T, Shimizu T: Stereotyped behaviors and compulsive complaints of pain improved by fluvoxamine in two cases of frontotemporal dementia. Seishin Shinkeigaku Zasshi 2006;108:1029–1035.
32 Chow TW, Mendez MF: Goals in symptomatic pharmacological management of frontotemporal dementia. Am J Alzheimers Dis Other Demen 2002;7:267–272.
33 Deakin JB, Rahman S, Nestor PJ, Hodges JR, Sahakian BJ: Paroxetine does not improve symptoms and impairs cognition in frontotemporal dementia: a double-blind randomized controlled trial. Psychopharmacology (Berl) 2004;172:400–408.
34 Anneser JM, Jox RJ, Borasio GD: Inappropriate sexual behaviour in a case of ALS and FTD: successful treatment with sertraline. Amyotroph Lateral Scler 2007;8:189–190.
35 Lebert F, Stekke W, Hasenbroekx C, Pasquier F: Frontotemporal dementia: a randomised, controlled trial with trazodone. Dement Geriatr Cogn Disord 2004;17:355–359.
36 Moretti R, Torre P, Antonelli RM, Cazzato G, Bava A: Olanzepine as a treatment of neuropsychiatric disorders of Alzheimer's disease and other dementias: a 24-month follow-up of 68 patients. Am J Alzheimers Dis Other Dement 2003;18:205–214.
37 Freedman M: Frontotemporal dementia: recommendations for therapeutic studies, designs, and approaches. Can J Neurol Sci 2007;34(suppl 1):S118–S124.
38 Caselli RJ, Yaari R: Medical management of frontotemporal dementia. Am J Alzheimers Dis Other Demen 2008;22:489–498.
39 Curtis RC, Resch DS: Case of Pick's central lobar atrophy with apparent stabilization of cognitive decline after treatment with risperidone. J Clin Psychopharmacol 2000;20:384–385.
40 Mendez MF, Lipton A: Emergent neuroleptic hypersensitivity as a herald of presenile dementia. J Neuropsychiatry Clin Neurosci 2001;13:347–356.
41 Pijnenburg YAL Sampson EL, Harvey RJ, Fox NC, Rossor MN: Vulnerability to neuroleptic side effects in frontotemporal lobar degeneration. Int J Geriatr Psychiatry 2003;18:67–72.
42 Kerrsens CJ, Pijnenburg YAL: Vulnerability to neuroleptic side effects in frontotemporal dementia. Eur J Neurol 2008;15:199–201.
43 Czarnecki K, Kumar N, Josephs KA: Parkinsonism and tardive antecollis in frontotemporal dementia – increased sensitivity to newer antipsychotics? Eur J Neurol 2008;15:111–112.

44 Fellgiebel A, Muller MJ, Hiemke C, Bartenstein P, Schreckenberger M: Clinical improvement in a case of frontotemporal dementia under aripiprazole treatment corresponds to partial recovery of disturbed frontal glucose metabolism. World J Biol Psychiatry 2007;8:123–126.
45 Moretti R, Torre P, Antonelli RM, Cazzato G, Bava A: Effects of selegiline on fronto-temporal dementia: a neuropsychological evaluation. Int J Geriatr Psychiatry 2002;17:391–392.
46 Adler G, Teufel M, Drach LM: Pharmacological treatment of frontotemporal dementia: treatment response to the MAO-A inhibitor moclobemide. Int J Geriatr Psychiatry 2003;18:653–655.
47 Rahman S, Robbins TW, Hodges JR, Mehta MA, Nestor PJ, Clarke L, Sahakian BJ: Methylphenydate ('Ritalin') can ameliorate abnormal risk-taking behavior in the frontal variant of frontotemporal dementia. Neuropsychopharmacology 2006;31;651–658.
48 Goforth HW, Konopka L, Primeau M, Ruth A, O'Donnell K, Patel R, Poprawski T, Shirazi P, Rao M: Quantitative electroencephalography in frontotemporal dementia with methylphenidate response: a case study. Clin EEG Neurosci 2004;35:108–111.
49 Andersen C, Östberg P, Wahlund L-O, Winblad B: Treatment strategies in frontotemporal lobar degeneration. Brain Aging 2003;3:3–6.
50 Reed DA, Johnson NA, Thompson C, Weintraub S, Mesulam MM: A clinical trial of bromocriptine for treatment of primary progressive aphasia. Ann Neurol 2004;56:750.
51 Allain H, Bentué-Ferrer D, Tribut O, Mérienne M, Belliard S: Drug therapy of frontotemporal dementia. Hum Psychopharmacol 2003;18:221–225.
52 Litvan I: Therapy and management of frontal lobe dementia patients. Neurology 2001;56:S41–S45.
53 Merrilees J: A model for management of behavioral symptoms in frontotemporal lobar degeneration. Alzheimer Dis Assoc Disord 2007;21:S64–S69.
54 Robinson KM: Rehabilitation applications in caring for patients with Pick's disease and frontotemporal dementias. Neurology 2001;56:S56–S58.
55 Talerico KA, Evans LK: Responding to safety issues in frontotemporal dementias. Neurology 2001;56:S52–S55.

Mario F. Mendez, MD, PhD
Neurobehavior Unit (116AF)
V.A. Greater Los Angeles Healthcare System
11301 Wilshire Blvd., Los Angeles, CA 90073 (USA)
Tel. +1 310 478 3711, Fax +1 310 268 4181, E-Mail mmendez@ucla.edu

Author Index

Subject Index